Praise for
What the Other Mothers Know

"The Mother of all mothering books. There's no aspect of childhood that this book doesn't cover—including a few you never even knew about."

—*Mariska Hargitay*

"This book is wickedly funny, shamefully honest, warm but not gooey, and smart but not convoluted. It is only slightly sardonic, and is 100 percent guaranteed bullshit-free. It doesn't talk down to women, it doesn't worship children, and in chapter 10 you'll find a recipe for the world's best chicken soup."

—*Camryn Manheim*

"I've always marveled at the other mothers and longed to be in their club. *What the Other Mothers Know* has helped me achieve membership status. This is a must-read for all moms. It's entertaining and funny, with valuable information. Order fast-food burgers for your child's class twenty-four hours in advance? Who knew? Okay . . . the other mothers did."

—*Lori Loughlin*

"If only I had read the part about the car upholstery and *especially* the high chair before I bought the really cool expensive ones with cloth snap-on seat covers that now look like the drop cloths in the monkey house at the Los Angeles Zoo!"

—*Peri Gilpin*

About the Authors

MICHELE GENDELMAN is a comedy writer, with credits on *Newhart* and *The Facts of Life,* among many other shows. A writer for animated series on Cartoon Network and PBS, she also teaches screenwriting and film history at Los Angeles City College, and is married to television writer/producer Andrew Guerdat. Her crowning achievement is having instilled a strong sense of humor in her children, Marc and Abby, and above all, teaching them to laugh at themselves. Marc and Abby, however, prefer to laugh at their mother. And so far as they're concerned, her greatest accomplishment is her mashed potatoes.

ILENE GRAFF is an actress and singer, best known for the six seasons she spent as the mom on the ABC television comedy *Mr. Belvedere.* Her Broadway stage work includes *Promises, Promises; Grease;* and *I Love My Wife.* She costarred with Glenn Close in a film version of *South Pacific,* and has appeared in miniseries and feature films; her CD, *Baby's Broadway Lullabies,* was nominated for a Grammy. Married to composer Ben Lanzarone, her finest production is their daughter, Nikka, who is a musical theater performer in New York. Ilene is shocked but grateful to suddenly be one of the "other mothers."

DONNA ROSENSTEIN is a television casting director in Los Angeles, currently working on *The Ghost Whisperer,* starring Jennifer Love Hewitt, and numerous other television and film projects. As a senior vice-president at ABC Television for many years, she oversaw the casting of such hits as *NYPD Blue, Roseanne, The Practice,* and *Twin Peaks.* She has worked with Oprah Winfrey, Sylvester Stallone, and the Muppets, but her most successful project to date is her sixteen-year-old daughter, Georgi. As a single mom, Donna juggles full-time work and hands-on parenting; has never missed a teacher conference, recital, or buying a pair of pointe shoes; and lives to tell the tale due largely to an entire village of "other mothers." She is thrilled to be able to pass along their sound, loving voice.

WHAT THE OTHER MOTHERS KNOW

WHAT THE OTHER MOTHERS KNOW

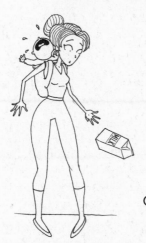

A Practical Guide
to Child Rearing
Told in a Really Nice,
Funny Way That
Won't Make You Feel
Like a Complete Idiot
the Way All Those
Other Parenting Books Do

Michele Gendelman, Ilene Graff, and Donna Rosenstein

HARPER

NEW YORK · LONDON · TORONTO · SYDNEY

HARPER

WHAT THE OTHER MOTHERS KNOW. Copyright © 2007 by Michele Gendelman, Ilene Graff, and Donna Rosenstein. All rights reserved. Printed in the United States of America. No part of this book may be used or reproduced in any manner whatsoever without written permission except in the case of brief quotations embodied in critical articles and reviews. For information address HarperCollins Publishers, 10 East 53rd Street, New York, NY 10022.

HarperCollins books may be purchased for educational, business, or sales promotional use. For information please write: Special Markets Department, HarperCollins Publishers, 10 East 53rd Street, New York, NY 10022.

FIRST EDITION

Designed by Nancy Singer Olaguera
Illustrations by Michael Ahern

Library of Congress Cataloging-in-Publication Data is available upon request.

ISBN: 978-0-06-113986-4

ISBN-10: 0-06-113986-6

07 08 09 10 11 ISPN/RRD 10 9 8 7 6 5 4 3 2 1

*We gratefully dedicate this book to the many mothers
who shared with us their stories and wisdom,
and above all to our children,
Marc, Nikka, Abigail, and Georgi,
whom we love more than words can express.*

Contents

WHAT THE OTHER MOTHERS KNOW

INTRODUCTION

The inspiration for this book came not from motherhood but from hamburgers.

A couple of years ago, Ilene's daughter was in a community theater musical production, and the proud mom invited her friend Donna to attend a performance. That night, Los Angeles traffic was the nightmare it usually is, and the only kind of bite they could grab before curtain time was of the fast variety. So they stopped at a nearby In-N-Out Burger, a California chain famed for its extra-meaty patties and old-fashioned chocolate shakes.

As they sat at a plastic table cramming Double-Doubles into their mouths, Donna told Ilene about something that had recently happened at her local In-N-Out Burger. And it was an experience guaranteed to strike fear into any mother's heart . . .

The week before, her daughter's third-grade teacher had called to ask if she would bring twenty-six hamburgers and twenty-six bags of fries to school the next day for their end-of-year party. And not from any old McGreasy's, either. No, these had to be from In-N-Out Burger, whose relatively healthy food preparation had earned this particular teacher's seal of approval. Donna knew that the treats a mom brings to the class can either boost her kid's playground "cred" or turn her into a social outcast, so she took the assignment seriously. So seriously, in fact, that she took the next day off to ensure punctual delivery of this very special meal.

That morning, Donna decided she'd use some of her free time to work out at the gym. But first she'd swing by her local In-N-Out when they opened at ten o'clock and put her order in early. Humming happily, she approached the paper-hatted youth behind the counter. "Hi. I'm going to need twenty-six hamburgers and twenty-six orders of fries for—"

Young Paper Hat gave her an apologetic look. "Uh, sorry, ma'am, but we're, like, understaffed today and we have a lot of, y'know, like, big orders to fill." (People in Southern California use the word "like," like, a lot. Y'know?)

Donna smiled. "Oh, that's okay. I don't need to pick them up now, I need them at noon."

"I understand, ma'am. But it's the last day of school and there are lots of, y'know, like, last-day-of-school parties, y'know? We won't be able to fill a noon order."

Donna turned pale and her heart dropped somewhere around the laces on her Nikes. "No, no, you don't understand. I have to have these burgers. I *have* to!" On the verge of hysteria, she asked to speak with the manager.

(As Donna told this tale, Ilene broke out into a sweat. It was either the suspense, or the onions on her Double-Double.)

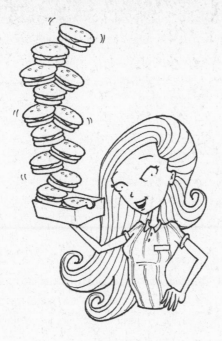

After half an hour of Donna's sobbing, cajoling, and outright begging, the In-N-Out manager finally realized that the only way he would get rid of her was to take the order. She practically collapsed against the counter with relief, and swore her undying gratitude.

When Donna returned at noon, she saw the manager handing out big boxes of burgers and fries to several women she recognized from school. They all looked so serene, like Buddhas with mascara and lip gloss. She stopped a mother she knew and asked what she'd done to rate such special treatment. (This was, Donna added, one of those know-it-all Über Moms, the sort who at seven in the morning is in the per-fect—and clean—Juicy French-terry sweat suit, with her hair blown out, wearing earrings.)

The other mom gave her a condescending smile and said, "What 'special treatment'? You just place your order the day before, and they have it all ready for you."

Ordinarily, Donna would've appreciated the irony of ordering fast food a whole twenty-four hours in advance, but she was too stunned by the mere concept of it. Never, ever would she have guessed that such things were possible.

"I mean, who would know that?"

Ilene sighed and squirted another dollop of ketchup onto her fries. "The *other* mothers know that. The other mothers *always* know those things."

Donna looked up from her chocolate shake in mid-slurp. "What the other mothers know . . . That's a book."

"You're right," said Ilene. "We have a book! Cool! What do we do first?"

Donna thought for a moment. "I think we find someone to write it with us."

A mutual friend told Donna and Ilene about a writer she knew whose daughter had attended the same school as Donna's and knew those other mothers only too well. They met with Michele at their local Starbucks to discuss the project (it was still a little too early in the day for burgers), and she agreed that this was a book whose time had come. A couple of decaf

Toffee Nut Frappuccinos later, the three women knew they were ready to write the mother of all mothering books.

The Other Mothers know all sorts of things. They know that enrollment for preschool begins the moment the EPT strip changes color. They know that bringing the coach Krispy Kremes will get their seven-year-old spaz his big shot at playing infield. And they know that principals can't tell the difference between the white polo shirts the school sells for $30 and the kind Target sells for five bucks.

What's their secret? Simple: they didn't become Other Mothers until after they'd been mentored by *other* Other Mothers—women with older kids, women who'd been up one child-rearing road and down another and still had the energy left to talk about it.

Of course, the concept of learning from Other Mothers is hardly a new one; consider the primitive societies of New Guinea, where the only people who know which animals and plants are safe to eat are the older women. But where do you get good information like that without being completely embarrassed? Lucky you: instead of having to consult a toothless hag in a smelly hut, all you had to do was walk into a store and buy this book.

But don't wait until you have children to start your Other Mothers network. Once you are, in the immortal words of Ricky Ricardo, "'spectin'," and you've found a good obstetrician, the second most-important item on your to-do list is not "Listen 2 Classical CDs 2 Make Fetus Brilliant" but "Make Friends w/ Women Who Have Young Kids."

If you don't have any friends or relatives with children, then seek them out at your office. In the grocery store. Stalk them in the park, if you must. Ask for advice, recommendations on preschools, and old maternity clothes. This network is called the Other Mothers Starter Kit.

We've benefited from it and now we've written this book to share and celebrate the wisdom of the Other Mothers who have helped us and our friends as we've raised our children from tots to teens—especially their advice on things we had absolutely *no idea* we were supposed to know how to do. We don't pretend to be professionals, like Dr. Spock or Dr. Phil; we're just three Dr. Moms, hands-on working parents who have to budget our time and our money. Online research and parenting magazines are fine, but there are some things you can only learn from the Other Mothers. And, after all, why reinvent the wheel when you could be off doing—oh, wait, you have no free time, you're a mother.

With four children of varying ages between us, we've jumped through just about every fiery hoop in the wonderful circus called Motherhood, and none of us could have done it without the Other Mothers. They were our safety net as we inched our way across the tightrope of the Toddler Years. They helped us juggle our kids and careers without dropping either one. And they taught us that while someone has to clean up after the elephant, it doesn't always have to be Mom.

Some of the information in this book is so simple and obvious that when you read it you'll want to kick yourself—just as we did when we first heard it. But we've also got that *other* advice that is so devious, so fiendishly clever that you will marvel at the minds behind it. Consider it a maternal E-Z Pass.

So, read on. May you be rewarded with some valuable tips, a bit of comfort, and more than a few laughs; every mother needs as much of all three as she can get.

Just beware that if you follow the advice of the Other Mothers, some day you'll be one too.

And sit up straight while you're reading, young lady!

1

Bringin' My Baby Back Home

You're nine months pregnant. It's down to the zero hour. You've checked off your list of things to do:

- Paint nursery
- Interview pediatrician
- Buy car seat
- Apologize to store manager for breaking water on aisle 5

So far, so good. But you forgot one little thing. Whether they're two minutes old or two years, babies are messy. Have you ever looked—*really* looked—at the backseat of a car where an infant has been riding for longer than five seconds? Milk contains calcium. What happens when milk dries? It leaves calcium deposits. Before you know it, the backseat of your lovely new cloth-upholstered Camry or Volvo wagon will look like someone coated it with ricotta cheese, then baked it with a blowtorch.

True, you can always hook your super-sucking Bissell 1200B SpotBot Hands-Free Compact Deep-Cleaning Carpet Cleaner up to an extra-long extension cord, and see if it reaches into the backseat. That'll be a neat trick while you're postpartum. Then how about taking it to the local car wash? Sorry, girls, but they won't get near Baby-Barf Guano.

What the Other Mothers Know

Buy or lease a car that's upholstered in vinyl or leather. Both materials are virtually indestructible, not to mention, leather just looks so darned cool. The leather package will set you back around $650 on a new car, but trust us, it's worth every penny. And did we mention that leather looks cool? It looks so cool, in fact, that your husband will probably go for it even without hearing about the increased resale value.

If your car is a two-door, you're better off trading it in for a four-door anyway. You won't want to have to bend and twist when you're still recovering from childbirth; between the sutures and sore nipples, just the mere thought of bending is an oucher. Later, as the baby gets bigger and heavier (they gain approximately twenty-seven pounds per day that whole first year—no, not really, it only feels like it), you'll practically break your back every time you put her in or take her out of the seat. Whether it's new or "previously owned," a four-door vehicle is indispensable for traveling in comfort after your baby arrives.

Does That High Chair Come in Leather?

We're not exactly biker chicks, but as long as we're on the subject . . . we decided that if we could've upholstered our entire homes in car leather, we would have. Because everything your baby does to the backseat of your car, he or she will do a million times more to your sofas, your chairs, your carpet—oh, heck, just go ahead and have the entire house covered in car leather.

What the Other Mothers Know

If your sofas and chairs are upholstered in fabric, see if the material can be Fiber-Sealed or treated with some similar type of stain- and dirt-repellent. If you are considering leather furniture, you'll probably want to go with finished leather, which has a top coat that will resist staining from liquids ("liquids" being the operative word here). Think of your baby as a puppy that doesn't shed, but drips.

Car Seats a Go-Go-Go

Okay, you buy the car. You buy the car seat. You and your spouse take the car seat out to the car with the instruction manual. You take one look at it and suddenly remember you promised your father that you'd organize Great-great-uncle Jasper's priceless collection of antique Moldavian fishing lures, and back you go inside the house, leaving the installation to your beloved, who is scratching his head in utter bewilderment at instructions that resemble blueprints for a space station. Unless you or your husband majored in quantum physics, you're going to waste the better part of a Saturday trying to figure it out—and your Saturday night arguing over whose fault it all was.

What the Other Mothers Know

Slipping some cash to the kid at the baby-furniture store to install and demonstrate how to use the car seat is the wisest investment you'll ever make. The Other Mothers also know that if yours is a two-vehicle family, you should keep a car seat in each one, so that you won't be constantly schlepping and reinstalling, schlepping and reinstalling. You can also tell whomever's hosting your baby shower that you need a car seat. (See below.) There's also nothing wrong with buying a "previously owned" car seat at a garage sale, so long as it's up to current regulations. Keep that one in the vehicle that your baby rides in the least. And if your parents or in-laws live in your town, pick up a third one for them too.

Baby Showers

So called because your friends and relatives shower you with presents of both the practical and frivolous sort, plus that third-trimester gift no girl can do without: a striptease by a George Clooney look-alike. You can register for shower gifts at national chains, such as Babies "R" Us, or give your shower hostess a list of items you'd be happy to receive.

But some women are superstitious about having a shower before the baby is born, much like they are about not announcing their pregnancy until the first trimester is over. What to do?

What the Other Mothers Know

Superstition aside, there are pros and cons to the pre- vs. postpartum shower debate. If you have the shower after you've given birth, you can enjoy a glass of champagne when the guests toast your beautiful new baby. Of course, since the baby is already here, you won't be able to join them, because that's the moment he'll pick to become hungry or need his diaper changed. And exchanging gifts won't be as easy to do with a baby in tow.

If the shower is held while you're still pregnant, you can't drink champagne; but no matter what you drink you'll be in and out of the bathroom ten times an hour getting rid of it, thanks to your fetus-mashed bladder. If something needs to be exchanged, you'll be the size of a Salt Lake City McMansion and probably won't fit between the seat and the wheel, but that's one of those times when husbands can come in handy. Our advice? If two friends offer to host showers for you, have one of them give you a shower *before* the baby's born, and the other, *after*.

If your hostess has never before thrown a shower, ask her to tell the guests that baby clothing in a variety of the bigger sizes—from ages 3–6 months on up to 18 months—is preferable to teensy-weensy newborn wear. Why? Because anything that's size 0–3 months will, typically, *not* fit a baby who weighs more than eight and a half pounds. Neither we nor any other moms we know can figure out where on earth this clothing is sized, but we suspect it's manufactured somewhere in Ireland, using wee leprechaun babies for models.

Items your baby will need:

- The Diaper Champ. This miraculous invention proves once and for all that God is a mom.
- Baby monitors. Every woman should have at least two sets, and one for her husband, too.
- A baby thermometer, nail scissors, and aspirator (trust us, this will save you a middle-of-the-night trip to the drugstore).
- A first-aid kit and handbook.

Items your baby can probably live without:

- The electric wipes warmer. Unless raising a *total wuss* is why you became a mother.
- The electric bottle warmer. What, do you think a starving baby will just sit there chatting patiently with you while the thing heats up? The old-fashioned way still works: placing it in a double-warmer on the stove top (remove with tongs).
- Cashmere onesies.

Other things you need to know about shower gifts:

- *Always save the receipts—and the boxes.* We guarantee that you'll buy or receive at least one item that doesn't work, one outfit that's too small, and something that just isn't right for your baby, which you'll need to return (the item, not the baby).

- If you receive duplicates of any items, don't take them back just yet; you might decide after the baby comes that having two bouncy seats—one for upstairs and one for downstairs—is ideal. If money isn't a concern, it's always better to have two of everything, especially for backup when something breaks.
- Don't laugh at that package of cloth diapers your tree-hugging friend gives you even though you've told her you're going to use disposables. Cloth diapers can be used a thousand different ways: to protect your "burping shoulder"; to dab at messy mouths; to clean up spills; as a makeshift bib; as a pad for the baby's head or tush when changing diapers away from home; and, when the baby has outgrown them, you'll find that they make the *best* dustcloths ever.

Are We Related?

Don't be disappointed when you behold your new baby and discover that you might not have given birth to the next model for the Gerber baby-food label. All newborns are funny-looking. Even yours. Often, especially yours. People laugh at newborns, and your little one will be no exception. Do not take umbrage.

What the Other Mothers Know

Instead, take a good, long look at those babies in the hospital nursery: fully one-fourth of their body is head, and a cone-shaped one at that; their faces are squished in; they don't have teeth or necks (well, no necks to speak of);

their legs are rubber parentheses; and because they don't yet know how to smile, that sober-as-a-judge expression they always wear looks ridiculous above a terry-cloth bib embroidered with "Spit Happens." You must understand that when people laugh at a newborn, they're not making fun of the child, but are making an unspoken observation: "Wow, some day this silly-looking, helpless little thing will be able to walk, talk, chew, read a book, throw a ball, drive a car, and produce more silly-looking, helpless little things." It tickles us to see infants, because what we're seeing is human potential in its purest, finest form. And when we're tickled, we laugh. So go ahead—if it doesn't hurt you too much to laugh—and yock it up at your baby's expense; trust us, she's too little to remember the dis.

Diaper Duty

Once you've given birth, you'll have a day or two in the hospital, where trained professionals are helping you to take care of the baby. During this time, you might want to pay attention to what they do, as Michele discovered.

I'd had a pretty rough delivery, so after my son Marc was born, I remained in the hospital for three nights. My obstetrician recommended I get as much rest as I could, and leave the diaper-changing to the nursing staff. No argument there. When we came home from the hospital, my mother and mother-in-law were there waiting for us, having flown in from the East Coast to help out. Marc started to cry soon after we got home, so I took him upstairs to his room to change his diaper. My first ever.

As my mother later described it, she and my mother-in-law were in the kitchen arguing politely over the best way to warm a bottle, when they heard me scream. They ran up the steps two at a time and found me leaning against the crib, horrified, pointing a trembling finger at the baby. "What did they do to him?!"

They just stared at me, totally bewildered.

"What, are you blind?!" I yelled. *"His penis is gone!"*

Then they started to laugh. And laugh. And laugh.

Michele

What the Other Mothers Know

A wet diaper can make an infant's penis retract to the point where it appears to be almost inverted.

After you've calmed down and realized that the nurses did not turn your adorable baby boy into an eight-pound, blue-eyed gelding, you will discover that diapering a little guy can be tricky at first—especially when you remove that warm, wet diaper, and exposure to the cooler air results in a one-gun salute that will, if his bladder is full, spritz you right in the kisser. Before you remove the wet diaper, have the fresh one unfolded and ready to go. Slide the wet diaper out from under him, then immediately place the unfolded fresh one over that loaded-and-dangerous frontal area. Now slide the underside of the fresh diaper under his tush, fasten the front as usual, and voilà—both mom and baby are dry!

Whether you're changing a boy or a girl, make sure there's no Vaseline, baby lotion, oil, or water on your fingers when you're using disposable diapers, or else you're sure to get some on the adhesive strips and then they

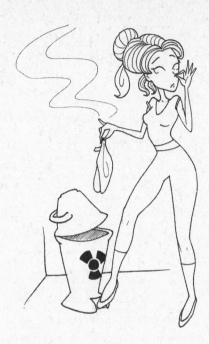

won't seal. To prevent this, keep a boutique-size box of tissues on or right beside the changing table so you can wipe off your hands before tackling motherhood's least-favorite chore.

Of course, you can avoid the diaper issue (no pun intended) by hiring a full-time nanny until your child's potty-trained. Never mind that you'll go into massive debt and your three-year-old will be standing outside the local nursery school some day holding up a sign that says, "Will recite ABCs for tuition."

Just Baby and Me

Your husband was able to take a few days off after the baby arrived, but now he has to go back to work, leaving you and the baby to your own devices. *No problem,* you say to yourself, *I can do this.*

For the first time, you and your child are alone. You gaze down at that perfect, beautiful little face . . . and then she starts to shriek like a banshee that just got its foot caught in a wood chipper. It is a moment of pure, stark, unmitigated terror unlike any you've ever faced before. "Nobody told me I was totally unqualified to do this!" you sob. Pretty soon you're crying even harder than the baby, your wails merging into one loud, dissonant duet.

What the Other Mothers Know

There's usually no mystery behind an infant's cry. They aren't yet old enough to be bored to tears, or feel the sting of jealousy, or shriek at a four-figure MasterCard statement. Babies cry because something's wrong in their tiny universe, and it is almost always physical: a wet or dirty diaper; hunger; diaper rash; gas; or they're over-tired. (Newborns can be overwhelmed by the strange new sights, sounds, and smells that confront them; haven't you ever been so over-stimulated that you couldn't fall asleep? If not, go hang outside Tiffany's window sometime and you'll see just what we mean.) Finally, the question we all dread: is the baby ill? Don't make the mistake many first-time mothers make, and feel guilty about "bothering" the pediatrician evenings and weekends. The reason they call it being "on call" is because the doctor is available to take parents' calls.

The first thing the doctor's office will ask is whether the baby has a fever, so before you phone, take the baby's temperature. The fact that most doctors' offices ask that this be done rectally might produce even more screaming, except this time it will be from you. Alternatives include the axillary, or armpit, method (often inaccurate by several degrees), tympanic thermometers (the kind you put in the ear, which most babies hate), the forehead strips (easy to use but not always accurate), and the pacifier thermometers (often accurate, but if the baby's used to her regular pacifier, she might hate this new plastic taste and ptooey it right back at you). You can try to make the more-accurate rectal method easier by laying the baby on her side so she can look at you, and distract her with her favorite toy for those two minutes it takes to get a digital reading. (Ask your pediatrician what method he or she prefers.)

There *is* one other thing that can make an infant cry, and it's the result of a mistake commonly made by new parents. Here, Ilene bravely admits hers:

*A*fter Nikka was born, my mother was here for about a week, then we had a baby nurse for another week. When the nurse left, I cried. What did I know? I didn't have any friends who had children yet; I didn't know anybody who had children, period. Nobody. Until this, the closest I'd ever come to being a mother was playing one on TV.

They left, my husband went off to work, and there I was, alone with Nikka. Suddenly she turned bright red, and began screaming. She broke out in little dots, and her skin was hot. I thought, *Oh my God, she's sick, she's going to die!* I called my mom back East, frantic. "The baby's burning up! I'm taking her to the hospital!" Mom said, "Wait a minute! Tell me, what's she wearing?" I told her, and then she told me what to do.

I slid Nikka out of her zip-up blanket-bag, then I removed her receiving blanket, her velour onesie, and her knitted wool cap and booties, and looked at her lying there in her diaper and sweat-soaked undershirt. She instantly stopped crying and focused instead on getting one tiny fist somewhere in the general vicinity of her mouth. She was absolutely fine. And I felt absolutely brainless!

Ilene

How was Ilene, or any other new mom, for that matter, supposed to know that babies run hot? And because Ilene also had one of those houses that are always cold, she'd automatically assumed that her fragile, delicate infant would turn into a kidsicle without all those layers. All Ilene needed was someone to tell her, because she just didn't have the practical experience to know any better. How grateful she was that she had that other mother—*her* mother—to set her straight.

On the Other Hand, There's That Much More of You to Love

Once you feel comfortable about leaving the baby at home with some responsible adult, or with his father, you'll be able to venture back out into the world. After being housebound for that first week after giving birth, fatigued from lack of sleep, and still a little tender physically, you'll either be dazzled by the size and scope of the world you'd forgotten once you started pushing, or you'll realize that the true center of the universe is that small bundle you left at home. Whatever your reaction, you'll be warmed by a new awareness that you are at one with all living things. Try to hold on to that feeling when you go to exchange the size 0–3 months clothes you received from the friend who did not heed your shower host-ess's suggestion and the cashier asks you, "So, when are you due?"

What the Other Mothers (and Fathers) Know

"Don't ever, ever ask a woman when she's due unless you're physically present in the delivery room and the baby's head has started to crown." (Hard-won advice from Ben Lanzarone, Ilene's husband.) Sarah Jessica Parker might be able to fit back into her negative-integer outfits a week after giving birth, but it's highly unlikely that you will, unless you have an entourage of personal trainers and private chefs. It'll take time, but you'll get there if you work at it.

One of the most time-honored methods for postpartum weight loss is nursing. The baby needs to gain pounds, you need to lose pounds; talk about a fair trade (and it's the last one you're likely to get from your child until she receives her driver's license and deigns to pick up a loaf of bread for you at the market in between her vital trips to the mall and her friends' houses). Other methods to trim the tonnage are enrolling in a postpartum exercise class, or taking the baby outdoors in one of those three-wheeled jogger-strollers: she gets to ride in style and comfort while you run and sweat (a nice metaphor for motherhood in general).

It's a Clothes Call

Perhaps, like many mothers who wish to raise their babies in as nonsexist a manner as possible, you've bought a bureau full of gender-neutral light green, yellow, and orange baby clothes. That's great. Just don't be insulted when strangers come up to you on the street or in a store and, after gushing and cooing over your new baby, ask, "Boy or a girl?"

What the Other Mothers Know

Unless you've slapped some lipstick on your daughter or a tool belt on your son, nobody can possibly tell the difference between a boy and a girl without looking in the kid's diaper, and no one wants to look in someone else's kid's diaper. If you anticipate being the sort of mother who's going to have a hissy fit at such questions, we offer this advice: if your baby's a girl, go pink and frilly. Whether you're Gloria Vanderbilt or Gloria Allred, every woman has dreamed of some day putting a real, live doll into the cutest, darlingest, most feminine little outfits and showing her off to a chorus of appreciative "oohs," "aahs," and "is-that-the-most-precious-thing-you've-ever-seens."

Because many infants lose a lot of their hair soon after birth (to remain smooth as eggplants until they're about a year old), another way to indicate a female is to put a girlie headband on her. Some are so ornate and froufrou that you could wrap one around a watermelon and people would exclaim, "My, what a beautiful baby girl!" Those headbands can, however, leave a temporary indentation on your baby's skin, so why make the kid suffer this early when she has a lifetime of dieting, moisturizing, and waxing ahead of her?

If your little one is a lad, blue is always a good "proud possessor of testicles" color, especially if it's denim. Better yet for identifying a man-child is clothing with any kind of sports or automotive theme. Nothing says "boy" louder than an infant-size sweatshirt with DALLAS COWBOYS across it, a sleep sack with basketball appliqués, or a NASCAR diaper cover.

Whenever you can, buy infant clothing in patterned material rather than solid colors; this will help to disguise those inevitable stains. Always wash infant clothing before you put the baby in it, to get rid of any dye or sizing chemicals that might irritate him. And be sure to remove all plastic tag-ties before you wash the clothes: that plastic string isn't much bigger in diameter than a hair, but if you've ever had one caught inside a seam of a sleeve, you know how sharp it feels. Against a baby's delicate skin? Wahhhhhhhh!

Lullaby Time

The only things babies do during their first few months of life are eating, eliminating some percentage of what they've just eaten, and sleeping. Newborns can sleep eighteen to twenty hours a day, although for some perverse reason they pick the middle of the night to be wide-awake.

When that happens, sing your baby a lullaby. That's why they're called lullabies: you lull the baby to sleep. But there's a trick to lullaby selection: you want only those songs that'll put your baby to sleep while still allowing you to remain in a sufficiently drowsy state so that you can conk out as soon as the baby does. Go for something with repetitive lyrics you don't have to think about and set up a mental playlist of songs that don't require any brainpower. We recommend doo-wop; a nice legato version of "Why Do Fools Fall in Love" always works, and will also serve to remind you how you got into this mess anyway.

We also recommend Ilene's CD, *Baby's Broadway Lullabies,* which is arranged so that the first songs are more active, and each successive song, quieter. By the time the last song plays, Baby is down for the count. And the second half of the CD is instrumental versions of the songs, so parents can sing along to the tracks or just enjoy the music. (Warning: don't play the CD in the car or you may fall asleep at the wheel.)

But when babies do sleep, you can use your "free" time to start applying to nursery schools. Just kidding. Not.

Whenever there's a baby in the house, we all go instinctively into tip-toe mode. While you don't want to play John Philip Sousa marches next to his crib, it's a good idea to get your baby used to the sounds of your house and your family. Dogs bark. Doorbells ring. Dishwashers rattle. If you make the baby's environment too quiet, he will be easily startled by everyday sounds later on, which will become a problem when you're trying to put him down for a nap or for the evening. Just as you need to adjust to having a baby, the baby has to adjust to living in your home.

What the Other Mothers Know

If you don't already have other children or adults or dogs making a racket in your house, get your infant accustomed to noise and plain old regular house sounds by keeping a TV, radio, or stereo on, set on low/normal volume, in whatever room she spends most of her time in. Just don't leave it on *The Sopranos,* or your baby's first words might be, "Yo, Paulie, ya [bleep]in' jamook, din I [bleep]in' tell ya ta whack that [bleep]in' [bleep]er already?!"

But We Have to Eat Too

Food is always an issue for brand-new moms. Not only the kind you give your baby, but the kind you make for yourself and your spouse. Before the baby arrived, perhaps you enjoyed cooking, sometimes spending an hour or more each night making some incredible, Rachael Ray–worthy meal you and your husband would savor every forkful of. After the baby arrives? You'll be lucky to grab enough time to slap a sandwich together.

What the Other Mothers Know

Give those pots and pans a rest for the first month or two. Instead of preparing meals, take that shower you haven't been able to find time for in the last three days, read a magazine, or just put your feet up while the baby naps.

If you don't belong to Costco already, buy a membership and send your husband off for their tasty prepared or frozen entrées. We're especially partial to those rotisserie chickens they're famous for, which literally cost less than what you could make them for at home. You can also purchase precooked foods from your local grocery store; most of the larger national chains and high-end markets now offer pretty edible items. Or order take-out. While takeout often isn't cheap, this is the period when you have to consider convenience and time; would you rather be spending that hour resting or being with your baby, or blanching baby vegetables (God forbid you should get so tired that you confuse the two)? About a month before your due date, make big batches of stews, soups, and pasta sauces, and freeze them in one-meal-size containers that you can thaw and heat in the microwave.

Take It to the Laundro-Mom

Don't worry about letting a few things pile up around the house; you'll get to them eventually. And if you don't, chances are they weren't that important anyway. Babies nap so their mothers can, too. Although you'll be tempted to do something useful when he goes down, like balance the checkbook or put a roast into the oven or stare at your boobs in the mirror and wonder how that set of 48DD's got on your body, you should do yourself, your baby, and everyone else in your family a big favor: get some rest.

However, if you're the active, compulsive type who simply can't sit still when something needs doing, there's always laundry. Face it: for the first six months of their lives, babies are little more than adorable, huggable, ten-pound extruders. (We call it the Three Ds: Drool, Drizzle, and Doody—sounds like a law firm in a Dickens novel.) Liquid in, liquid out, which means there will be laundry, laundry, and more laundry. And not just the baby's clothes, either, but every item of clothing belonging to anyone in the house who feeds or holds or changes or gets within projectile range of your effluvia-hurling bundle o' joy.

There is, however, such a thing as overdoing it.

*W*hen you have a baby, you wash his clothes separately, in mild Dreft, instead of using regular laundry detergent, right? Being the totally neurotic first-time mother I was, I sterilized everything, cleaned and washed everything by the book. My little boy is now three and a half. The other day my sister was over while I was washing his clothes in Dreft, and she looked at me as if I was insane. "You stop washing their clothes in Dreft when they're six months to a year old, for Pete's sake." I had no idea. No one told me. It was such an "I should've had a V-8" stupid moment. I still get ticked off when I think of the time, water, and money I could've saved!

Barrie
high-school teacher

What the Other Mothers Know

Wash your baby's clothing separately from yours, in Dreft, Ivory, Purex, or some other brand of mild soap designed specifically for infant wear. But after the baby's a year or so old, move up to regular-strength laundry detergent and throw his clothing into the same load as yours. All toddlers get dirty, whether from spilling food and juice on themselves, or crawling around on the floor. The more mobile they become, the filthier they get.

Set aside any poop-spattered outfits (your baby's and yours) and soak them separately in a plastic bucket of warm water and a squirt of grease-lifting dishwashing liquid. (The same properties that enable it to lift grease off of dishes enable it to lift poop off of cloth, thereby reducing the likelihood of stains setting.)

Wash your baby's clothing in hot or warm water, but use the delicates cycle. Baby clothing is washed far more often than adult or kid clothing is, so the less agitation, the longer the garments will last.

Crybaby!

No one likes hearing a baby cry, because we instinctively want to tend to the baby's needs and make him comfortable, happy, and peaceful. When a baby starts crying at certain social events or gatherings, a courteous parent removes the child to care for him in another room (see chapter 8 for more on this).

But there's little you can do when your baby starts crying onboard a plane. Where would you take her? Outside? Hardly an option, since those dumb airlines refuse to carry parachutes small enough. It never fails, either: your baby will scream or fuss during a flight *only* if you're seated next to a man who hates kids. Usually an unmarried, unattractive, nasty man, which might explain why he's unmarried and will probably stay that way. But one of our gal pals came up with a nifty Other Mother tip when this happened to her:

O̶ur son David was just seven weeks old when we had to fly from Miami to Omaha for my father-in-law's funeral. My husband had been up most of the night before, so I wanted to let him get some sleep. There I was, at thirty thousand feet, with my grieving, exhausted husband asleep next to me, and David started to cry. I tried giving him a bottle, I walked up and down the aisle with him, I changed his diaper. Nothing helped.

But that wasn't the problem. On my other side was a thirtysomething man, whose pudgy midsection, pale skin, and plastic pocket-protector screamed "computer nerd," one of those guys whose social life is playing video games or IM-ing other nerds about science mistakes on last night's episode of *Stargate-1*. First he said, really irritated, "Can't you do something about that baby?" Excuse me, *that baby*? I tried, but David kept crying. *Then* the guy rang for the flight attendant and complained that the baby was "creating a disturbance"!

She gave him a look (I could tell she was a fellow mom), then offered to find him another seat; except all the aisle seats were taken. So, I thought fast: I got the guy a set of headphones, paid for the movie, and bought him a drink. Thank God the movie was *Lord of the Rings, Part III*. He had two rum-and-Cokes, without so much as a thank you or even a smile. At least it shut him up and kept him off David's case. The man was such a total jerk. I only hope he never becomes a father.

Samantha
architect

We only hope that if he ever does, he gets twins. With colic. Who really hate flying.

Infancy is tough, but it is finite.

Your baby won't always be up all night, or go through forty-seven loads of laundry each week, or make messes in his pants (well, some males never do stop that but eventually it'll become some other woman's job to complain about).

But neither will he ever again grip your finger for the first time, or lift his head to look at you for the first time. At some point during that second or third month, your baby will begin staying awake a little longer during the daytime, and will be more alert when he is. He'll follow your movements with his eyes, wearing that solemn expression that all tiny babies have before they learn how to smile. And then one day, when you least expect it (there are about a thousand "least expect it" moments when kids are little), as you're smiling and making silly mom faces at him, he'll smile back at you. And when he sees you smile back in response, he not only becomes the world's worst ham, but something starts to hatch in his tiny baby brain. *Hey,* he thinks, *that got a response! Let's throw the big lady another one and see if I can wangle a trip to Toys "R" Us outta this . . .*

So just enjoy each and every moment of your child's babyhood, because she or he will never be a baby again. You'll probably never have a twenty-four-inch waist again either, but babies are a pretty good trade-off. Besides, your children will always think you're the most beautiful woman alive, no matter what size you are.

2

"Take Good Care of My Baby"

There comes a time when you must leave your child in the care of someone else. There's just no getting around it.

Some of you new mothers may feel that it's one thing to leave the baby with someone because you *have* to, but that it's another altogether to leave her with someone because you *want* to. Maybe you and your husband would like a meal out, just the two of you. Or perhaps you'd like to see a movie, or meet a friend for lunch. Or maybe you just need a few hours' respite from the rigors of new-mommy-hood. "What? Leave my baby so that I can enjoy myself? No, that just sounds wrong!"

It's perfectly normal to be reluctant, concerned, and downright terrified that whoever watches your child will turn out to be the Rebecca De Mornay character from *The Hand That Rocks the Cradle* or, at least, not do quite as good a job as you do. "Will she remember which one's his naptime blankie and which one's his night-night blankie?" "Does he know how to warm the milk properly?" "Does her parole officer know she'll be out past midnight?"

What the Other Mothers Know

Never feel guilty about leaving your baby in the care of someone who's capable and trustworthy. You're entitled to time off. Without it, you'll be too exhausted to be of much use to yourself or your baby.

The only time to worry is if your husband's arranged for his buddies to watch the baby in return for high-def ringside seats to the world heavyweight boxing championship courtesy of the brand-new fifty-six-inch plasma TV you didn't know you ordered.

Grandmas Are a Girl's Best Friend

For most of us, the people we trust most implicitly with our new baby are our own parents, especially good old Mom. Nine times out of ten, the best, wisest, and most practical child-rearing advice you'll ever receive will come from your mother. Never mind if it starts off with such groaners as "If you ask me . . ." or "Well, back in *my* day . . ." or the all-time classic "Not to tell you what to do, but . . ." (which, of course, means "Not only am I going to tell you what to do but I'm going to check and make sure you've done it, and you'll thank me for it").

For some of us, unfortunately, turning to Mom for help and solace is not an option. Sometimes Mom has passed on, or perhaps her health has declined. With so many women waiting longer and longer to have children, the chances are greater that when they do have a baby, their best, most reliable, and most caring Other Mother won't be around.

But if you're lucky enough that yours is still living, resides near you, and, most important, didn't screw *you* up too much when you were a kid, turn to Mom for babysitting. Unless your mother is a sexy sexagenarian on the prowl for Husband Number Two (or Three, or Four—we've all known a Holly Do-Not-Go-Gently-Into-That-Good-Nightly in our day), odds are she'll be desperate to spend just as much time with her new grandchild as she can anyway. In fact, it's commonplace to see grandmas provide the childcare for working mothers, and, sometimes, they even get paid for it. (Talk about an ideal situation: you get the best care ever *and* you keep your mother off the streets.)

What if your mother isn't available but your mother-in-law is? Aw, what the hell, give her a buzz anyway. At least she's free. Besides, she must've done something right to have raised the guy you let impregnate you. (Unfortunately, for the rest of her life your mother-in-law will steadfastly refuse to acknowledge that you contributed twenty-three chromosomes to this child—unless he turns out to be a serial killer or something equally heinous, and then she'll insist he inherited everything from *your* side of the family.)

What the Other Mothers Know

If you have both grandmas, or better yet, all four grandparents in town, you thank your lucky stars, dearie. Doting grandparents can sometimes be a tad too doting, but you shouldn't have to worry about the possibility that they'll spoil your baby. For starters, half the time they do it because they feel they shortchanged their own child (that would be you or your husband) and want to make up for it somehow, so please, take the opportunity to enjoy their discomfort. But really, when a baby is tiny, is it actually *possible* to spoil him? How exactly does *that* work? "Oops, I came into her room as soon as I heard her crying. My bad." "Damn it, I knew I should've held back when he wanted that bottle!"

Should there be an issue among the elders over who spends more time with the baby, here's how to dispense wisdom like Solomon *and* solve your weekend babysitting worries in one fell swoop: your folks get her every Friday night, and your husband's folks have her on Saturdays. Joint custody for grandparents!

The Babysitters Club

But what if you have no relatives or friends in the area, with baby know-how? Whom can you rely on, then, if you need a sitter?

What the Other Mothers Know

Don't expect to find babysitting for free. If your child is truly the most important thing in your life, shouldn't you expect to pay more for a babysitter than you pay to the guy who cleans out your gutters every fall? Call a licensed, bonded sitting service; there are dozens upon dozens in every metropolitan area. The women on their lists are, typically, single ladies from age twenty-five to seventy, who work a regular job during the day but want to pick up some extra income from sitting nights and on weekends. A woman who's always free Friday and Saturday nights probably isn't going to be the best-looking gal in town, but you don't want to be another ex–Mrs. Jude Law anyway. Expect them to be experienced, mature, and professional; and figure on paying anywhere from $2 to $5 per hour more than a teenager would charge.

But if you want to try the more traditional neighborhood babysitter, believe it or not, the phrase "responsible teenager" is *not* an oxymoron.

*W*hen Nathan was born, we were fortunate to have both sets of grandparents living in the area. But when he was around six months old, my dad was transferred upstate, and my in-laws retired to a community fifty miles away. We had to find a reliable babysitter if my husband and I ever wanted to spend two seconds together, so we asked around the neighborhood. It turned out there was a very sweet sixteen-year-old girl right down the street, with loads of experience. The problem was, she didn't have any Red Cross training, and there was no way I'd let anyone who didn't know CPR or the Heimlich maneuver watch my baby. So it was back to Friday and Saturday nights at home.

When I complained about it to my mother—silently cursing the day my father got his new job—she told me to just pay the girl to attend a Red Cross class in CPR. Of course! There was a Red Cross class offered at our neighborhood elementary school on Saturdays; so I paid Sarah the $5 an hour she charged for sitting, and four hours later she had her certificate and twenty bucks. My husband and I could go out knowing that

Nathan was in safe hands, and Sarah remained our babysitter through her high school and college years. I rate this advice as possibly the best my mom ever gave me, right up there with her subtle suggestion that getting a rose tattoo on my butt when I was nineteen was something I might possibly regret later on.

Delia
homemaker

In any case, if you and your husband wanna play, you gotta pay.

To Work, or Not to Work, That Is the Question

Making the decision to go back to work after having a baby is one of the toughest a woman can face, along with "Should I get bangs?" Some women choose to stay at home because their spouse earns enough money to support the family comfortably; they are fortunate. Other women who choose to stay at home do so despite the fact that their income will be missed, but they're willing to compromise and sacrifice; they are brave. Still others would love to stay at home but they need to earn money; they are the rest of us. Each decision brings its advantages and disadvantages.

For many women, it's not a decision, because the word implies choice. For most of us, there *is* no choice. We need to pay for those little incidentals, like food, mortgages, car insurance, etc. This is why more than seventy percent of mothers of young children in this country work outside the home. The days when the average middle-class American family could survive on one income are, sadly, over.

And to make the decision even more painful, some of us work in fields in which our careers would be pretty much over if we took even six months off to spend with our kids, much less six years. In certain fast-paced professions (stock brokering, investment banking, advertising, etc.), they'd have your name scraped off the office door before your obstetrician yelled "Push!"

What the Other Mothers Know

Whatever your reasons for returning to work or for staying at home, guess what? You don't have to give a reason. That's like saying you have to justify your decision to buy the blue twin-set instead of the green. This is a decision you make for yourself, with your husband. Don't let your parents, in-laws, self-help books, friends, colleagues, or even Oprah sway your judgment. Do what works best for you, what feels right for you, your family, and your situation.

Don't ever feel guilty because you have to, or want to, go back to work; and don't ever feel stupid because you're staying at home.

Split the Difference

Okay, so you've given birth, you've had your three months or six months at home with your child, and now you're ready to return to your job. If you haven't yet lost all your pregnancy poundage, you'll need a new wardrobe of work duds. Some women find that their shoe size changes after pregnancy; better pick up a few new pairs of Prada while you're out shopping. Oh, and you'll need one other little thing: child care.

Being a working mom is not easy, but there are ways to increase your chances of surviving.

What the Other Mothers Know

One very elementary tip is something we read years ago, when the actress Sally Field was asked how she coped with being a single, working mother: "I make longer lists, and I drive faster." We don't advocate

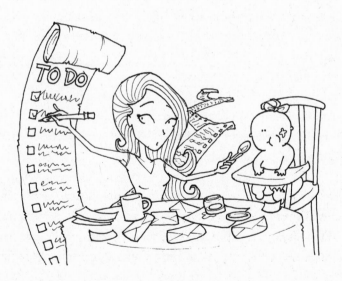

driving faster, but making lists goes hand in hand with being any kind of mother, especially one who works outside the home. Keep a pen and a notepad everywhere—your bedside, the kitchen, even the bathroom, and most of all, in your car. A retractable pen is best, so you don't risk ruining a blouse or hitting a telephone pole while you wrestle to put the cap back on a felt-tip.

And we don't care what the 3M Company says, we *know* that Post-its were invented by a mom.

If your husband's an actively involved papa, here's something you can do together for day care that will give each of you more time with your child:

I took several months' leave after Justin was born. Brad and I wanted to spend as much time with him as we could, but were in no position to quit our jobs and be stay-at-home parents. During my leave, we visited day-care centers, with disappointing results: too many kids, not enough personalized care, and not very clean. Then a friend told us about an in-home day-care provider who lived just three blocks from us. She was licensed, with fifteen years experience, and had space for one more baby. We fell in love with her, and so did Justin.

But we still wanted more time with him. After a quick trip to human resources, I learned that my company would allow me to work four days a week with full benefits, as did Brad's. So I arranged for my work week to run from Tuesday through Friday, and he arranged for his to run from Monday through Thursday. On Mondays, I was home with Justin; on Fridays, Brad was home with him. That way

Justin was in day care only three days per week, and the other two, he was home with one of us. Sure, we could use the income we lose by not working a fifth day, but spending time with our precious little boy is something that can't be measured in dollars and cents.

> *Karen*
> *IT manager*

Lactation, Lactation, Lactation

And now that you've returned to work, you'll have something new and challenging to deal with besides being a new parent: lactating in a place of business. When you're a host organism—sorry, a mother—it's got to be done, if you want your child to Eat at Mom's.

What the Other Mothers Know

Use the speakerphone while you pump your breasts. You can express yourself to your client while expressing your precious bodily fluid to take home to your baby (most cell phones as well now offer a speaker function). When you're finished pumping, label the contents and either refrigerate it or put it in a thermos to take home, where you can then freeze it for future use. If you're sharing a refrigerator with other employees, you might want to place the containers in a paper bag to head off the many breast "jokes" sure to come your way. And here's another tip: buy the cheapest bottles for freezing the milk, then put "quality" nipples on them when you're ready to feed.

No matter what your career or what rung of the corporate ladder you find yourself on, take comfort in knowing that many a CEO has attended meetings, brokered deals, and chewed out underlings while her breasts were leaking like sieves, or, as we like to say, many a silk blouse has taken a milk douse. Pack plenty of pads, and always be sure to keep some in your briefcase.

Yessir, She's Back in Business

Suppose you gave up your job so you could be home full-time with your child. Now that your "baby" is walking, talking, and solving algebraic equations, it's time to return to the wonderful world of work. You send out your résumé, or you sign up with a headhunter. Here come the interviews. Now how do you find a mother-friendly work environment? In most instances, asking a prospective employer if he or she is amenable to your taking time off to spend with your child, or bringing the child into work with you, will be met with a resounding "Next!"

Is there a way to scope out kid-friendly bosses without putting yourself on the line? Yes.

What the Other Mothers Know

One of the best working-mom tips we've ever heard came from a working dad. He happens to be a television writer, a profession in which the hours can be extremely long, but his advice applies equally to virtually any industry:

*W*henever you're interviewing for a job, look for photos of young kids on the boss's desk. If they're not all yellow and faded—the photos, not the kids—then this is a guy you want to work for, because he wants to get home at a reasonable hour to be with his family.

Casey

television comedy writer

Michele's son was a third-grader when she interviewed for her first television job. But she didn't need to look for kids' photos, because when her prospective boss stood up from behind her desk, she was clearly six months pregnant. Michele got the job, and every day that season she was home by six p.m. During the show's second season, Michele became pregnant with her daughter (must've been the water). By that time, the producer had had her baby and was herself learning the challenge of being a working mom. With newfound sympathy for the rigors of that last trimester, she insisted Michele lie down for half an hour every afternoon, whether she wanted to or not. Michele would have her siesta, then waddle back into the office refreshed and ready to tolerate yet more cracks from the other writers about her resemblance to Shamu.

Alternative Day Care

If you want to work without spending more on child care than you're earning, you have to find someone or some place that will do a good and affordable job looking after your child. There are day-care centers out there, of course, and we're going to assume that if you pursue that option, you'll do the basic legwork to make sure the one you choose isn't run by a sleeper cell.

But here are some alternative ideas for child care.

What the Other Mothers Know

Day care does not have to be expensive. Or even cost anything at all, for that matter.

I was still in college when Cody was born, and between paying tuition and not bringing in any money, day care was not in the budget. Meanwhile, a woman at my husband's office had recently had a baby and wanted to go back to work part-time; she also knew a stay-at-home dad who was looking for day care too. So, we decided to form a day-care co-op, and brought two more families on board, with each of the five families being in charge of care one day per week. No one wanted or needed full-time care, so we decided our "hours of operation" would be from eight thirty a.m. to one p.m. Most important, we shared the same ideals: we wanted a nurturing environment where trustworthy caregivers would be responsive to the needs of our kids.

Leaving five babies of varying ages in the care of one person was too big a job, so we had two parents working daily. If something came up and a mom or dad wasn't available on their day, we were fine with grandparents or aunts and uncles filling in. We kept the arrangement until Cody started kindergarten, and it couldn't have worked out better.

Laurie
accountant

Co-ops are a great way to save on child-care expenditures, but if you can afford it, there's another option to think about, as this young mom discovered:

*W*hen my first son was born, the magazine I worked for allowed me to write at home. I hired a woman to take care of Ethan in our house twenty hours per week, which was ideal. Until Ethan started to crawl, that is. Once that happened, and he knew where Mommy was "hiding," he was not happy until he'd found me; and then he wouldn't let the sitter get near him. I realized I'd have to start working at the office again, but I didn't want to put Ethan in a day-care center; nor could my husband and I afford daily, full-time help in our home.

My neighbor two doors up, who had a little girl eight weeks older than Ethan, was in a similar situation and couldn't afford full-time care at home either. Worse, the wonderful part-time housekeeper she'd had for years now needed full-time work and would be leaving as soon as she found it. When I commented that it was too bad we couldn't just shove our houses and our kids together and make one forty-hour work week, the thunderbolt struck us both at the same time: what if Estela worked for our two families full-time, taking care of both babies instead of one? Half the week she'd watch our babies at my house, the other half, at Sandy's, and when the kids were napping, do what cleaning and laundry she could. Sandy and I would each pay half of her full-time wages (with extra thrown in, since caring for two babies at once is hard work). Estela took the offer and started immediately. The kids love her, we trust her implicitly, and for half of every week, at least, my house doesn't look like a cyclone blew through it.

Leslie
journalist

By being open to new ideas and by pooling their resources, Leslie and her neighbor got the help they needed, the housekeeper got the full-time employment and salary she wanted, and the children were kept in a familiar, comfortable environment that was convenient to all.

Working

Running a business out of the home is something that many mothers do, to varying degrees of involvement, until the "baby" is old enough to go to school. But for those five years until then, working at home can be problematic, with or without day care. Especially since a determined youngster can track down a trying-to-work mommy like Davy Crockett in diapers.

What the Other Mothers Know

Our opinion (which you obviously want to hear or you wouldn't have bought this book) is, when you're at work, you're at work, and when you're with the baby, you're with the baby. Putting the two together is like mixing oil and water and expecting it to turn into salad dressing, when all you'll end up with is a bowlful of soggy lettuce.

Okay, so maybe the metaphor doesn't work. But if *you* want to work without feeling torn about leaving your little one, go for a job with a company that offers on-site day care. Among the Fortune 500 companies to include such perks are General Mills, IBM, Wachovia, Eli Lilly, Nestlé, Sony, Johnson & Johnson (boy, had they better!), and many, many more.

Come to Papa

But there's one other form of inexpensive and reliable child care that even the experts often overlook.

What the Other Mothers Know

Husbands!

First off, let's assume your husband's not one of those men who think Pull-ups are something you do in the gym.

Some of us are incredibly lucky to have husbands who want to be involved in the raising of their child (and if you have half a brain, you'll *stay* married to them). So, make sure you give your guy a turn at the business end of the baby.

And while we're on the subject of dads and kids, we have some words of wisdom to share from our friend Barbara Williams, admissions director and assistant head of the Village School in Pacific Palisades, California. Once a year, she does a special Dads Night, when only the papas are invited to discuss their child-rearing questions and issues openly. This is what she's learned:

> *I*n the five years I've run Dads Night, virtually every father's biggest complaint has been, "My wife doesn't trust me to take care of the baby, and then she gets mad when I don't help."
>
> It's a very valid point, which moms need to listen to. Your husband or your partner loves the baby every bit as much as you do, so does it really

matter if he feeds her peas instead of carrots? Does it really matter if he puts him into the blue suit instead of the red suit? The important thing is, you need to trust Dad; he's not going to let anything happen to the baby. If you really want to have a true partner in child-raising, you have to trust him and let him be a father.

Of course you should let your husband take care of the baby, whenever possible. Besides, babies love beer.

Aw, we kid the menfolk. Some moms insist that no matter what you do, your husband will never be as responsible or as dedicated a parent as you are. Don't you believe that for a second. If your man doesn't know what he's doing but is willing to learn, remember that the only way he *can* learn is by doing.

And guess what often happens when a mom calls her office to say she has to stay home with a sick child? "Oh, these women," grouses the boss, "always putting their kids before their job." And, "No wonder women can't get ahead in business, they're always taking time off to take care of their kids." Well, here's something you can do to appease the workplace gods:

*D*on and I were at wits' end when Alissa came down with a cold one evening. Even though it was nothing serious, we wouldn't be able to take her to day care, because they don't have a sick room. Worse, my boss was already on the warpath about the number of days I'd taken off for mommy duty. But Don, on the other hand, hadn't missed a day in three years, so, we thought, *Why not let* him *ditch a day?* Sure enough, not only was Don encouraged to stay home with Alissa until she got better, his boss actually felt guilty because *he* never spent enough time with *his* kids.

Joan
office manager

When a *man* calls in to say he has to stay at home with a sick baby, everyone gushes, "What a great father he is!" "Such a role model!" "Gee, is his wife a lucky gal or what?" So, why not use him?

Just a Spoonful of Sugar

Everyone's heard of the best-selling book *The Nanny Diaries,* although we think that any nanny who had enough time to keep a diary probably wasn't a very good nanny to begin with. But these days, you don't have to be super-rich to hire in-home help.

Usually when you invite someone into your house, it's because the family is visiting, or you're throwing a party, or you're having something repaired. Hiring a nanny, whether to live out or live in, is all three: she's sort of a family member, sort of a guest, and sort of a kid repairman. Obviously, it's an important decision, so here are the three words to live by: get references, duh.

But here are a few additional tips we've picked up over the years.

What the Other Mothers Know

You don't have to go to an expensive agency with some hoity-toity English-sounding name that's supposed to make you think of Mary Poppins.

Sometimes the best referral comes from someone you know personally. For example, if you know a family with teenagers who've outgrown their nanny, you don't have to go very far to check out her work: look at the kids! Are they out sitting on the hood of their car with a bottle of malt liquor and a carton of jumbo Grade-AA throwin' eggs? If not, you might want to take her résumé.

Another good way of finding a nanny or housekeeper is to scout your neighborhood.

> When I was pregnant, I knew I'd need to go back to work fairly soon after the baby came, so, by my eighth month, I was desperate to find help. One day, on my way home from the office, I noticed a big house around the corner, with a for-sale sign, a tricycle, and a slip-and-slide in the front yard. I put two and two together: big house, family with kids, in escrow . . . equals Nanny Up for Grabs! Totally on a whim, I rang the doorbell, and the wife answered. Just as I'd thought, she and her husband were moving to another city and their nanny would soon be looking for work. I met Carla right then and there, and when the family did move several weeks later, I wound up with a proven child-care wonder, and, as Carla always laughs, she didn't even have to learn a new bus route.
>
> *Felicia*
> *sales representative*

Donna found her nanny through the nurse she employed the first month after her baby was born. The nurse had a cousin, who had a friend, who had a sister with child-care experience who was looking for work. Sixteen years later, she is still with Donna, even though the "baby" is almost ready to drive herself to school. We refer to this method as the unofficial Nanny Network: put the word out on the grapevine and it works better than Craigslist.com. Sometimes faster, too.

Many new moms are convinced that when they hire a housekeeper or nanny, they must have someone young. The reasoning tends to go, "Sure, my baby might sleep eight hours a day *now,* but when he's six months old he'll be a real live wire. And once he starts crawling, he'll need someone who can keep up with him."

*B*y the time my daughter Hillary was walking, we knew that this kid would tire out the Energizer Bunny. So I hired a woman in her early twenties, who I felt would be able to match her pace. And she did. For about six months. Then she decided to become a full-time college student, and I was back to square one. So, the next time out I hired Anna, who was in her late fifties. She may not have been able to get crazy in the sandbox for three hours straight, but she was patient, experienced, and I even think her grandmotherly vibe helped Hillary calm down a bit.

Bonnie
computer consultant

Something else to remember about nannies is that their presence in your child's life is finite. Sooner or later they will retire, or quit to have children of their own, or start a business that we'll all wind up working for some day, so, little Todd will have to learn to live without his beloved nanny (for whom he's already no doubt created an adorable nickname).

Somehow, though, this inevitable transition seems more natural and less abrupt when the caregiver is an older woman rather than a younger one.

An issue that many new moms face after they've hired a full-time housekeeper or nanny is feeling like the nanny's become a member of the family. But as long as you're writing their paycheck every week, they ain't family. No matter how fond your children are of the caregiver, they are *your* children and it is *your* house.

> *W*hen we hired Sylvie, I thought we'd really lucked out. She was French (but not a "babe"), college-educated, enthusiastic, and my son Eric totally adored her. In fact, he adored her so much that my husband and I ended up bending over backwards so that Sylvie could spend as much of her time as possible with Eric. Well, pretty soon we found ourselves making her breakfast, unloading the dishwasher, vacuuming. And then one day, as we were folding sheets, we looked up at each other and practically said at the same time, "Why are we doing *her* laundry?" So we had to sit down with Sylvie and reestablish our employer/employee relationship—starting with the idea that *she* was the employee.
>
> *Debra*
> *public-relations executive*

Before you hire a housekeeper or nanny, look over her letters of reference and her CPR-training certificate. Then, meet with her and specify the duties you'll expect her to perform. This is especially important with nannies, many of whom come to this country from Europe, where there is a strict "class" division between those who care for children and those who do housework.

If you're wealthy enough to hire both a nanny and a housekeeper, lucky you; if you can afford "only" one, however, find a woman who can both take care of the baby and do the housework. (Remember what they called that kind of woman back in the day? A wife.) This person should be able to:

- Follow the baby's schedule (feeding, naps, etc.)
- Play with the baby
- Take the baby for walks
- Bathe the baby
- Do laundry and ironing
- Clean the house
- Prepare meals
- Work overtime if you need it (if she can, set an hourly rate *now*)
- Be available via cell phone (if she doesn't have one, get her one)
- Do the weekly marketing. If she takes the baby with her, you must provide a car seat for her vehicle and cash for gas. Xerox a copy of her driver's license and go to your state's Department of Motor Vehicles Web site to check her driving record. (You'll also want to see proof of insurance.) If she's driving your car, make sure she's covered under your policy.

It's better to go a little overboard on the expectations rather than downplay them, because no employee, no matter what her line of work, appreciates having extra, unanticipated duties added to her job after she's started. If, later on, you see that the housework is too demanding, either lighten her duties or, if you can afford it, hire a cleaning woman to come in once a week to do the heavy housework (while reminding the housekeeper that this is only a *temporary,* stopgap measure). Of all the people in your life you least want seething with resentment, it's the woman who's caring for your pride and joy. Nope, the only woman who should ever resent you is your mother-in-law, for stealing her son.

After one enterprising New York mom hired a nanny, she created a Web site called HowsMyNanny.com; each parent who registers pays a fee and receives a tag to hang on her stroller, similar to those "How Am I Driving" bumper stickers you see on trucks. If a caregiver is seen publicly mistreating or neglecting her young charge, a watchful passerby can log onto the Web site and make a report. There might be such a service available in your area; if there isn't, you might consider starting a Web site of your own. Just remember, when *you're* the one pushing the stroller, you could get busted too.

No matter whom you choose to watch your child when *you* can't watch your child, no matter how much research and preparation you do, rest assured there will be separation anxiety. Not the baby's; yours. Babies have their own problems to worry about, like trying to shove their foot all the way into their mouth.

MORE OTHER MOTHERS' TIPS

- Check the bulletin board at your local supermarket, where teenagers and retirees often advertise their babysitting services.
- Ask friends, neighbors, and colleagues if they have teenage daughters or nieces who babysit; even if they don't, they might have friends who do.
- Call the career placement and planning office at your local college or university and ask for a list of students who babysit.
- Interview your local bonded, insured babysitting service so that you might have emergency "backup" in case your regular in-home day-care provider is absent.
- Contact the nearest day-care center—whether your baby is enrolled there or not—and ask if any of their employees sit at night or on weekends.
- Pretty teenage babysitters end up dating, and soon you and your husband won't be. Find a plain girl, or a religious girl whose parents won't let her even look at boys until she's forty-seven.
- Plenty of teenage boys babysit too! Better to have a responsible lad than a girl who puts the safety pins in her nose instead of in the diaper.
- Whether you file the long or the short form, if you work, you can be eligible to claim the child-care tax credit; speak with your accountant.
- If you have a pool and a nanny who doesn't know how to swim, hire a swimming instructor for both her and your child.

IT'S IN THE BAG

When your child is age six months to two years, the following items should be with you at all times:

- Disposable diapers
- Baby wipes
- Bottle of milk
- Pacifier
- Teething ring
- Floaties or other water-safety equipment
- Cheerios
- Stuffed toy
- Play toy
- Bibs (for drool-proofing the baby's clothes)
- Cloth diaper (for drool-proofing your clothes)
- Change of clothes (for you and the baby)
- Ziploc baggie (you'll find out why in chapter 3)
- Cell phone, with pediatrician's number on auto-dial
- Wallet
- Keys
- Hairbrush (not that you need one, because after the baby was born and you realized blow-drying was not on the schedule, you started going to Vin Diesel's barber)
- Cosmetics bag (because you'll have approximately thirty-seven seconds to apply makeup at red lights en route from home to your destination, we recommend concealer, lipgloss [easier than lipstick to apply without looking], mascara, and a little atomizer of perfume to mask the lingering aroma of sour milk and old apple juice)

3

~∽~

"Baby, We Were Born to Run"

(or "Morris, Just Move the Lladros Already!")

"I turned my head for one moment and . . ."

We all know what comes next.

". . . before I knew it, she rolled off the changing table!"

And you thought carpeting the baby's room was merely a decorating choice.

Babies are pretty tough; in fact, most of them will bang their noggins more often than a metalhead at a System of a Down concert, and still live to tell the tale (which is more than some System of a Down fans can say). Never forget that babies are adventurers. Their job is to make their way through the physical world, learning how stuff works. That talcum powder on the changing table is just a container of talcum powder to you, but to your crawling nine-month-old it's something with endless possibilities. "Ooh, it smells nice and stuff comes out of it in poofs when Mom shakes it!"

And then that baby lightbulb comes on. "Hmm, that stuff inside is white. Let's see, milk is white, and I love milk, so . . . let's RO-O-O-O-OCK!"

What the Other Mothers Know

Just like they say in every child-care book ever written, your baby will suddenly become capable of performing life-endangering acrobatics before you know what's hit you (and he's hit the floor). He can't talk yet, right? So, what do you think he's going to do, announce, "Hey, Mom, look what I can do" before he executes a triple-gainer out of his crib?

Probably the most common time for a pre-crawler to test his wings is when you're changing him, because you're busy reaching for wipes, diapers, etc. So here are two ways to prevent a changing-table tumble:

- Keep all the products you need—diapers, powder, ointment, wipes—within arm's reach
- Install safety straps if your changing table or area does not have them already

Here's another method for keeping your little wiggle-worm from swan-diving off the changing table: attract the baby's attention away from all those tempting objects by placing a mobile or a big, colorful photograph directly over the table—either mounted on the wall above it or taped up on the ceiling itself. If posters of a scantily clad Shakira or Jessica Alba can keep a sophomore's eyes glued to the ceiling in his dorm room, a nice Little Miss Spider or Winnie the Pooh cutout should do the same for your six-month-old.

While it's always convenient to have a changing table, you can use a dresser top for this as well (and they're a lot cheaper). No matter what you use, however, be sure that you install safety straps.

If you have a two-story home, you should also consider having more than one changing area, so that you're not racing from upstairs to downstairs a gazillion times a day. If you have a downstairs bathroom large enough, place a second changing table in there. (If money's tight, buy a "previously owned" changing table at a garage sale or on eBay.)

Drop and Give Me Twenty Yards

Crawling is quite possibly the cutest thing a baby does, right after smiling, and making that priceless "thbbbbbbb" raspberry sound with attendant lower-lip blubber-flutter. When babies crawl, they look like big, chubby cartoon crabs scuttling across the floor, ready for action; unfortunately, they don't come with a shell. At the top of their list of priorities is following Mom, Dad, and any family pets wherever they go, and that means up the stairs, down the stairs, and right into the kitchen, where your husband just dropped a soda bottle that promptly shattered into a million tiny pieces all over the floor.

What the Other Mothers Know

Tip number one: tell your husband to buy his Coke in cans.

If you can't sprint like a steroid-juiced Olympian after a speedcrawling youngster, then you'll need gates. There are two places where you should always have them: at the top or the bottom of the stairs, and at the entrance to the kitchen. There are lots of books and Web sites out there that can show you where to purchase these handy gadgets and install them.

Now, for the tips they *don't* tell you . . .

If you've been considering recarpeting, or redoing your hardwood floors, wait until *after* your child starts walking and is able to do so competently. You won't believe how tough little kids and their gear can be on floors and rugs: the playpens, walkers, play "yards," Big Wheels, pull toys, and other stuff they throw, drag, and bang on the floor can scuff all but the toughest-material flooring (yes, titanium is impervious to scratches, but will it go with chintz?). If your hardwood floors were installed or refinished before the baby started crawling, and you want the most painless way to protect them, buy some big, cheap area rugs and throw those down where your baby does most of his or her playing. We're partial to the Isaac Mizrahi designs at Target, where a fabulous, stain-resistant eight-by-ten-foot area rug can be had for around $250.

Carpeting is lots softer anyway for a baby to motor on, and it's relatively easy to keep free from, uh, organic buildup, provided you steam-clean it on a regular basis. For $200, you can purchase a steam vacuum (with a 20 percent off coupon from Bed, Bath & Beyond or Linens 'n Things, it's only $160). Or you can shell out around $7 a day to rent a Rug Doctor or similar steam vacuum from your local supermarket. But whether you buy or rent a steam cleaner, try to con your husband into handling this chore. While the newer machines are much lighter and easier to push than they used to be, why should you have to struggle with it, you delicate little thing, you? Actually, we have the perfect idea for getting husbands to actually *want* to vacuum, but for some reason Harley-Davidson won't go into the home-cleaning business.

If you own valuable area rugs or Oriental carpets, there is only one way to protect them from children: put them in storage for the next four years. (We meant the carpets, but if you're tempted to pack the kids in there with them too, we understand.) Have the rugs professionally cleaned, roll them up, and stow them somewhere they won't get mildewed or provide a hundred generations of moths with an all-you-can-eat buffet. When your child is old enough and no longer deliberately dumps sippy cups full of grape juice on your floor to watch the pretty patterns, it'll be safe to bring the rugs out again and display them in all their woolly glory.

Some babies don't crawl so much as they scoot across the floor on their tushies (just beware of rapidly shifting diaper contents). A scooter's clothes will wear out much faster in the back than a crawler's do, so put your scooter in corduroy or denim pants or overalls; they'll wear longer and better, and their seams are reinforced.

What Goes Up . . .

One of the things babies do after they've learned to crawl—but before they learn to walk—is to stand up. It's awfully cute to see them in a vertical position after they've spent the previous ten months or so lying down or sitting. Finally, they're looking more like miniature humans instead of something that might've crawled out of a pod in a 1950s sci-fi movie. But there's one aspect to standing that you might not be aware of.

My daughter Bryn had recently learned how to stand, by grabbing the bars of her crib as they all do and pulling herself up. One night I'd just put her down after her eleven o'clock feeding and gone into my room when I heard her crying. There she was, standing up in her crib, tears streaming down her little cheeks. I laid her back down, went back to my room, and two minutes later she was standing up and crying again. Well, this went on for an entire hour! Finally, at the end of my rope, I called my mother in Indiana, where it was three in the morning. I told Mother what was happening and she said, in this groggy voice, "Sweetheart, she doesn't know how to sit back *down*. Show her how to bend her knees. Good night." And that's exactly what the problem was. I showed Bryn how to do it, she practiced it a few times, and she got it. As she curled up with her blankie, she gave me this grateful expression that said, *Now I can hit the hay, Mom. Thanks!*

> Diane
> *magazine editor*

What the Other Mothers Know

"What goes up must come down" doesn't describe only gravity. A simple physical movement that an adult has done ten thousand times is a brand-new experience for a baby, requiring her to use a hitherto untapped set of little muscles.

You'll see this happen earlier in your baby's development when he's around four to six months old and is able to rest himself on his forearms while lying on his tummy. He'll crane his head up and around to check out the action, happy as a miniature frat boy at a spring-break kegger. And then that big fat head begins to feel heavier and heavier, and in ten minutes he'll be crying like a frat boy with an empty keg, because he doesn't know how to rest his noggin on the floor or his arms. What you can do is lie down on the floor right beside him and demonstrate how to roll over onto his back, like a turtle, only the other way around.

The same thing happens when a crawler/toddler—let's just call them crawdlers—tries to climb back downstairs after negotiating his or her way up to the second floor of the house. They don't have a built-in reverse gear. So when they get stuck, you get up on those stairs right along with them and just show them how to do it.

Oh, and never worry about calling your mom for advice in the middle of the night. When there's an opportunity to show her daughter that there's something she knows more about, never mind that you interrupted her erotic dream about being examined by Dr. McDreamy.

Safety First, but Not for Five Figures

Child-proofing.

One mother's opinion is that child-proofing has become a high-end industry only after nannies became more affordable to the middle class. She says we have to child-proof because we're afraid the nannies aren't watching the kids as closely as they should be. Whatever the reason, many parents get ripped off by the ever-growing army of so-called consultants. That four-figure Superdyne All-in-One Turbo-Charged 3000 Radon

Early Warning Kit, E. Coli Detector, and Video Surveillance System they want to sell you? It's probably a little bit more than you need to maintain baby's safety.

What the Other Mothers Know

Baby-proofing is important, but it's not an excuse for not watching the baby. As another of our friends says, "Don't just child-proof the house, house-proof the child."

But here are some other tips that will help you deal with your child's growing mobility.

(Incidentally, just in case you inadvertently missed an outlet or a cupboard door, don't be afraid to say "no" to a one-year-old who's ventured dangerously close to the verboten area or object. Use the Stern Mommy Command voice accompanied by the Stern Mommy Face, pick her up, and physically move her to another spot until you get the problem fixed. Yes, she'll cry. Not because she'll be scared, but because she'll think Mommy is mad at her. And yes, you'll feel awful, but this is exactly what our forebears meant when they'd say, "This is going to hurt me a lot more than it hurts you.")

Do:

- install electrical outlet covers.
- install gates at staircases and doors leading into a potential danger area, such as a kitchen or a bathroom.
- install latches on any cabinets containing toxic cleansers or medications. Duh. (Moms who reside in Earthquake Country should

consider keeping those latches on permanently, so that bottles of meds and supplies won't fly out of the cabinets and shatter during a tremor.)

- put up clear acrylic sheets across French doors and low-hung windows, so your little one won't run through glass. Once he is older, remove the sheet, then inform your husband that you have to repaint the room because of the nail holes. And new paint simply *has* to be followed by new furniture.
- pool owners: install a floating or side-mount alarm that blares like a maximum-security prison klaxon when a child gets anywhere near it; and make sure that fencing around the pool and your property is built to code.
- if you have swinging doors, install hook-and-eye latches to keep them stationary until the baby is old enough to understand two-way traffic.
- put night lights where a crawdler cannot touch the hot bulb.

Don't:

- let yourself be convinced by "professional" baby-proofers who do things like measure the gaps between vertical slats in an outdoor fence and warn that anything wider than a human hair will result in an AWOL toddler. Go online and check your state's building code to learn the recommended width.
- let doggy or cat doors stay open if your crawdler is small enough to wriggle through.

- invest in a video baby monitor until you've checked with your computer consultant. If your house has wireless, or you network several computers via a router, it can interfere with the monitor's reception.

Coffee tables and other furniture with corners are always a nightmare for parents of toddlers, which is why companies are making millions off of selling corner cushions, those soft plastic bumpers that fit around coffee tables. Or you can do what this mom did.

When Julie was around a year old and just starting to walk, she bumped her head on a corner of the coffee table we had in our living room. I immediately went out to buy edge bumpers, but the directions said the adhesive backing could ruin antique furniture. Well, I'd inherited this table from my grandmother and I was not going to risk ruining it. So I put the coffee table into storage, which is where we kept it until Julie was three.

Susan
elementary-school teacher

Susan gave us another good tip on baby-proofing: if you hire a consultant to baby-proof while the baby's still tiny (or not even born), you don't yet know whether you have a "climber" or not. You will know soon enough, however, if the baby starts trying to rocket-launch herself out of her crib, so consider waiting to see what type your baby is before you invest in heavy-duty "anti-climbing devices."

Babies cannot resist the temptation to pick up anything that looks play-with-able, edible, or breakable. Keeping them away from things they can destroy or hurt themselves with can be a daunting task.

*W*hen my son Marc was a toddler, and my first husband and I flew back East from California to see family, we visited his aunt Rae and uncle Morris, who lived in New York, surrounded by a collection of Lladro figurines they'd been acquiring for years. Their only son was in college, and they didn't have any grandchildren, so the Lladros were scattered about the living room, within hideously easy reach of a curious toddler. Marc was lurching into everything like Frankenbaby, so the moment we walked into Aunt Rae's and I saw that throng of figurines, I panicked. So did my husband, my mother-in-law, my father-in-law, and most of all, Uncle Morris. After twenty minutes of us alternately grimacing and jumping up like jack-in-the-boxes to stop Marc whenever he toddled near an expensive "tchotchke" (Yiddish for "tiny knickknack, big price tag"), Aunt Rae finally gave Uncle Morris a look and said, "Morris, just move the Lladros already!" That became my standard line for whenever we had to baby-proof an area in our own house, or in someone else's when we were visiting: "Morris, just move the Lladros already!"

Michele

Other things that crawdlers will make a beeline for are DVD players and VCRs, which are typically placed on a shelf below the television set. Unfortunately, it's inconvenient to move a DVD player or a VCR out from beneath a TV, because the wiring can be complicated and difficult to reach. If it's your baby and your house, buy a TV cabinet with doors

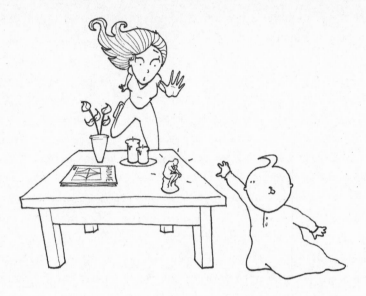

that include knobs or pulls that can be latched together. If your components are open-access, buy VCR and DVD-player guards. These are clear,
unobtrusive acrylic panels that attach by adhesive over the front panel of
the components to prevent kids from pressing buttons. If you do not take
these precautions, then you must make sure someone's always keeping an
eye on the baby when he's in that room, or the next time you want to watch
Dirty Dancing and do a little sofa mambo with the hubby, you'll discover a
handful of half-masticated pretzel rings jammed in the loading slot.

Another thing crawlers cannot stay away from is an eye-level roll of
toilet paper. Here's a tip from Michele's husband, writer Andy Guerdat.

I was watching TV when I heard this mysterious "whuppida-whuppida" sound. By the time I tracked it down, our daughter Abby, who was then about eleven months old, had managed to TP our entire bathroom floor. After spending half an hour trying to get the paper rolled back onto the cardboard tube, I gave up and threw out a perfectly good roll of Kimberly-Clark's finest. As I was putting the new roll on, it occurred to me that from now on we should simply make sure the toilet paper feeds off the *back* of the roll rather than the front. That way Abby could make her new spinny toy whuppida-whuppida to her heart's content, but the paper stayed in place. Until she figured out a way to do it backwards.

When you're visiting people who don't have children, you cannot expect them to reconfigure their furniture and possessions to suit your crawdler. However, a considerate host understands that the best way to keep a toddler away from valuable items is to put them out of the child's reach for the length of the visit, *before* the child arrives. So, call ahead when you can, and ask your hosts to put the crystal vases and the knickknacks on the top shelf of the china cabinet.

Port-a-cribs are handy not only when you're going out of town to visit and will be sleeping over, but when you take the baby with you *in* town.

*A*fter my daughter Ashley was born, the only way I was ever able to get my hair done for the next two years was to shlep her and her port-a-crib to the salon. Since I was a client of long standing, and the salon had lots of floor space, I'd set the crib up near my hairdresser's station, and Ashley would play happily with her toys while I got colored and cut. Since the majority of hairdressers and their clients are female, there's always a multitude of moms and would-be moms around to help keep the little one entertained.

Cassandra
actress

Obviously, you don't make an appointment with Jonathan Antin or Frederic Fekkai and bring your nineteen-month-old along in a playpen, but if getting a sitter during the daytime is difficult for you, call your stylist in advance and ask if bringing the baby in a pen would be all right. (If your baby does end up making a fuss, leave an extra-generous tip afterwards, and don't bring the baby with you to your next appointment or you might end up with a Marge Simpson 'do.)

Incidentally, an unexpected benefit Cassie discovered from her experience was that when Ashley turned three and was ready for her first haircut, she was already comfortable enough around Cassie's stylist that she allowed her to cut her hair without a peep—more important, without Cassie having to endure the traumatized toddlers at one of those children's salons. If your child's a girl and starts whining for more, be firm and say, "Sorry, toots, but the only highlights you're getting is the magazine at the doctor's office."

Round Up the Baby Posse!

You've not only got to watch your own youngster when he's mobile; sometimes when people come to your home, they'll expect you to watch theirs as well.

*W*hen I was five months pregnant with my second child, some friends came over on Christmas. I had been up until three a.m. Christmas Eve, assembling toys for Kari, my three-year-old; gotten up in time to see her open them; prepared breakfast and Christmas dinner; and then, as most of the guests were leaving and I was ready to collapse, these friends showed up. The mom sat down and started chatting with my mother, and left *me* to chase after her eighteen-month-old daughter, who started by taking a glass ornament off the Christmas tree and beating it on a giant tin of cookies! Then she went after all of Kari's brand-new toys, and after breaking one of those, decided she could have even more fun terrorizing the cat, who finally retaliated by scratching her. (Hey, here's a lesson: pull the cat's tail and he may scratch you!) My friend got incredibly indignant about it, as if it were the cat's fault! It was horrible.

Gabrielle
mortgage broker

What the Other Mothers Know

When a lazy visitor waltzes in with a toddler in tow and sees it as an opportunity for free day-care, do what Gabrielle learned to do: just look her in the eye and say, "Oh, gosh, my house isn't really baby-proof anymore"—even if it is. Your guest will get the message and watch her little monster like a hawk the whole time she's there. There is a strict etiquette and protocol on this subject that should be followed to the very letter, as if it were a State Department edict and every mother an ambassador: when you visit someone who has children, do *not* expect her to watch yours.

Don't Be a Pill

One of the places you least want your baby nosing around in is a purse. Some babies will do anything for money, and it's always tragic when good kids resort to stealing. Especially when they're not even potty-trained.

No, really, it's because a purse might contain prescription medicine, and folks who are taking meds for this and meds for that sometimes carry a veritable pharmacopia. Does your mom take anti-statins for cholesterol, and routinely keep a pillbox in her fanny pack that she sets within reach on the kitchen table? Does your visiting brother-in-law have Lamisil for his toenail fungus in the suitcase he leaves wide-open in the guest room?

Now, you certainly shouldn't start sniffing purses and luggage like a German shepherd at the airport. Nor do you have to butt into others' business ("Honestly, Sis, with that jerk you're married to I'm really surprised you're not taking a much stronger antidepressant than this one"). All you need to say to your guest is, "I'd hate for the baby to ruin whatever you might have in your purse," and they'll be so nervous about having their condoms or AARP membership card trotted out in public you won't have to worry about putting it out of the way.

Hey, I'm Walkin' Here!

As thrilling as it is to see your child walking, it opens up a whole new world, a world of sharp objects and hard surfaces. And the more your child walks, the more you'll find yourself sounding just like one of those dazed eyewitnesses on CNN when they describe an alligator or wild-bear attack: "Dear God, who knew that they could move that *fast*?!"

Your job as a mother is not only to care for your child but to protect him. It's up to you to do that in such a manner that your toddler negotiates his way through the world with a sense of adventure tempered by common sense. It's only natural that your little boy should want to race over to that shiny, bright-red fire engine parked down the street; you have to see that he gets there without jay-toddling on his way.

It's only reasonable, then, that parents find some means of restraint that permit their wandering toddlers to poke about the world while keeping the world from poking into them.

What the Other Mothers Know

The best way to restrain your child is by staying close: hold on to your child's hand at all times. Or carry your child. If you're expecting to do a good bit of walking, then bring the stroller along (keep a smaller, umbrella type stroller in the trunk of your car at all times). If you're going into the market, put your child into the seat of the shopping cart instead of letting her walk with you. (And now that all the bigger grocery stores carry those cart-sanitizer wipes when you walk in, slip a few extra into your pocket for cleaning your trunk.)

Another method some moms use is a wrist leash or body harness. These items have engendered a considerable amount of controversy. Those parents opposed to the leash feel it conveys a negative impression to the child; it suggests that the use of a physical restraint rather than words to keep a small child in line is, well, humiliating. Those in favor of the leash argue "better safe than sorry."

No matter where you stand on the Great Leash Debate, just acknowledge the plain and simple fact that *no parent* is capable of keeping an eye on her child every single second as she walks through a mall or down a grocery aisle; only a cyborg could do that. But you might want to think twice before becoming the Mom-inator:

Someone told me about this new gadget called a wireless toddler leash, where the parent carries an electronic receiver, and the transmitter is attached to the child. If you're suddenly separated by more than ten feet or so, the alarm goes off. It sounded like a great idea to me, because I've never liked the concept of leashes. So, the next time I took Jeremy to the mall, I used the wireless leash. Unfortunately, as we were leaving, Jeremy darted ahead, and this horrible screeching went off. It scared Jeremy so much he burst into tears, and everybody around me thought I'd been caught shoplifting! After spending the next ten minutes trying to calm Jeremy down and convince store security that I'd paid for my lingerie, I decided to be a low-tech mom again.

Shelley
professor

Well, here's a radical suggestion, and it's even more low-tech than hand-holding: if at all possible, how about *not* taking your child to the mall or the grocery store, and leaving him at home with Dad or Grandma or the sitter instead? After all, isn't three a little young to be learning how to comparison-shop? Besides, when your kid turns twelve, you won't be able to pry her loose from the mall, so why push it?

(And Moms, we believe we speak for all humankind when we ask you to please keep your sick child out of public places whenever you can. Yes, it's lovely that you want to share little Madison's microbes and bright-green runny mucus with us, but we think little Madison might be more comfortable at home—we know *we* will be.)

Keep It Clean . . . or Maybe Not

Babies are messy, no doubt about it. They make even your husband look like Felix Unger. And once they start to crawdle, they're able to spread the dirt all throughout the house. You want to keep things clean and neat, but not to such an extent that it ends up driving you, your child, or the rest of your family completely, utterly insane. There'll be time enough for that when your kid becomes a teenager.

Baby wipes were the first wipe invented, probably by a mom who was using a wet nap on a toddler's greasy hands after a visit to Kentucky Fried Chicken and had a brainstorm about the other end. Over the years, wipes have sprung up for every possible part of your body or house: now we have wipes for granite, for stainless steel, and there's even something called the Field Towel, a "Giant Full-Body Wet&Dry Towel" (slogan, "This is *not* your Mama's baby wipe!") that's used by soldiers in the field (and they get almost as dirty as toddlers).

What the Other Mothers Know

Regular baby wipes aren't handy only for the tush-al area; they can clean up a multitude of other sins as well, if you find yourself short of other wipes. They can clean hands and faces, and car seats. They can remove chocolate ice cream from shirts. And Ilene also recommends them for makeup removal on the run; the ones with moisturizer are especially kind to the delicate eye area. Just don't make the mistake our friend Patty did, and use them to clean CDs!

Is there such a thing as too clean? One of the things Michele appreciates most about her mother-in-law, apart from having raised the greatest husband and father who ever lived, is her attitude toward germs and dirt. (Was that a shameless bid for a piece of jewelry or what?)

Children develop natural immunities that last a lifetime by encountering germs when they are little. In my opinion, keeping things sterile at home will not allow them to build up antibodies to fight those germs when they run into them (and they certainly will) in the big, wide world.

Lyn
retired RN

A friend of Ilene's (who has begged for anonymity in case her children should ever read this book when they become parents someday) had a real thing about germs. For a while.

When my first child dropped a pacifier on the floor, I'd pick it up and sterilize it in the dishwasher. With my second child, I'd pick it up and rinse

it off under hot running tap water. After my third came along, I'd just spit
on it and hand it back!

> *Mary Anne*
> *homemaker (Oops. Sorry about that, Mary Anne!)*

We like the five-second rule: if it falls on the floor but you pick it up
in less than five seconds, it's technically not dirty. That's a rule that was
definitely invented by a mom.

According to the Hygiene Hypothesis, a new theory making the
rounds of the medical-research community, infants' and kids' immune sys-
tems may not develop as well if they are not exposed to certain common
irritants. The theory goes on to say that because 90 percent of the country's
population now lives in suburbs and cities, distant from farms, farm critters, and their accompanying bugs, we've become a lot more susceptible to
such things as dust; dust mites; pet dander and saliva; and pollen. So, if you
don't vacuum every day, don't clean up after your pets, leave food-covered
dishes in the kitchen sink at night, allow leftovers to turn a lovely sage-
green in your fridge, and keep your windows open, it's still possible your
kids will grow up just as healthy as those whose parents maintain homes
sterile enough to perform surgery in.

The sacrifices we mothers must make for our children . . .

Puttin' in the Dog

There's nothing sweeter than watching a faithful dog follow the child of
the house, cleaving protectively to the side of its wee master. It causes our

hearts to swell with love and admiration for Man's Best Friend and his millennia-long devotion and dedication to our species.

What the Other Mothers Know

Oh, get real. Dogs don't follow crawlers and toddlers because they want to watch out for them. They follow them because they want to eat whatever *food* the babies drop on the floor.

If you have a dog, put that mop and vacuum cleaner away. Fido will be thrilled to do the job for you. And if you have a two-story house, get two dogs and assign one to each floor!

But remember, crawdlers and dogs are about the same mental age, so be careful that yours doesn't go after the dog's dish. Ground beef lips probably aren't on the pediatrician's list of recommended foods. Besides, the one thing that could cause even the most lovable pooch to snap at the most adorable baby is Alpo-poaching.

He Who Has the Most Toys Wins

Crawdlers will pick up one toy, play with it for two minutes, then discard it to pick up a new toy, play with that one for two minutes, and on and on. It's just a natural by-product of their overwhelming curiosity. But by the end of the day, your family room will resemble the warehouse in the final scene of *Citizen Kane*.

It's exhausting to pick up after a toy-crazy child, but this new mom has learned a good way to get around it.

*W*hat I do is put all Holdenn's toys away at night, so in the morning it's just bare floor. Then, I place a small selection of toys into each of these various stations we've set up around the family room: I put some in the playpen, some in a basket in one corner of the room, and some others in a toy box in another corner of the room. Then, throughout the day, as Holdenn rotates, the toys rotate with him. You can't spend all day worrying about the clutter, or, worse, picking it up all the time. But this way when he does clutter up an area, it's confined to that one area. Otherwise, yeah, it probably would drive me legally insane!

Lianne
realtor

Other mothers we spoke with about this had learned to keep some sort of toy bin handy in virtually every room their crawler or toddler spends time in; just like having more than one changing table if you live in a two-story house, having additional toy bins will also spare you added trips up and down the stairs. Or, better yet, you can start teaching your crawdler that her toys belong in her room, and use a wagon or favorite toy vehicle for one of the storage bins.

*M*y daughter's toys started taking over the house when she was around two. We figured it was time for Katie to start learning that her room is the proper place for her toys. She loved going shopping with me and had one of those plastic Fisher-Price shopping carts, so just before bedtime each night, I taught her to go "toy-shopping": we'd go through the house picking up her toys (or at least some of them), stack them into the cart, and take them to the "store" (her room). So far it's worked pretty well, except for when we go to Toys "R" Us and I have to explain that it works just a little differently there than it does at home.

Rhonda
homemaker

Out of the Bottoms of Babes

One of the dirtier trails that babies leave behind is, well, what comes *out* of their behind. Poopy diapers. Arghh! But one of the more wonderful inventions to hit the baby-products market is the Diaper Champ. It truly is amazing how it compacts the, uh, matter and turns it into a tiny, easily-disposed-of packet. And because it retails at around $30, virtually anyone can afford it. But what do you do if you're going out with the baby, or going off to visit someone who doesn't have a baby—or a Diaper Champ—in the house?

What the Other Mothers Know

Invest in gallon-size Ziplocs for disposing of the disposables when you're away from home. If their zip-ability keeps the air away from the food, it'll keep the smell out of the air. At the end of your visit, deposit the offending bundle from your bundle of joy into your hosts' garbage cans, and no one will be the wiser. Except for maybe the garbage man on Tuesday morning.

I Shoulda Stayed in the Crib

You'll know your child is too big for her crib when you're feeding her breakfast one morning and she says, "Mommy, you think Letterman will ever get another shot at hosting the Oscars?"

Usually, though, you'll know if your child is climbing out of bed at night, because you'll hear that distinctive thud-scamper-patter. And, of course, she'll want to waltz into your room and show off her latest contusion. Time for a big-kid bed!

What the Other Mothers Know

If your three-year-old is reluctant to bid bye-bye to her beloved crib (and the fun and adventure of "going over the wall"), you might try this as a way of getting her with the new nighttime program:

Stacy grew out of her crib when she was twenty-nine months old. But she didn't quite grasp the concept of her dad dismantling "Cribby," and when she saw our cleaning lady take it away for her newborn, she howled, poor kid. I had no idea how on earth we'd get her to sleep in the junior bed we got her, but then I remembered that sneaky way my mother always used to get me to do something when I was a kid: by making it seem as if it was my idea. So I took Stacy to Bed, Bath & Beyond and told her she could pick out any bedding set she liked. She chose a comforter that had sailboats all over it, and she fell asleep in her new bed without a problem. Maybe the comforter worked a little too well, though; she's fourteen now and still takes it with her on sleepovers.

Wendy
attorney

We Live Here Too!

One last thing to bear in mind as your child begins to move upward, outward, and every-ward, is that it's just as important to make your house as baby-*friendly* as it is baby-proof.

Reserve one of the bottom cupboards in your kitchen to hold lighter-weight pots, pans, and lids that your crawdler can play with. Anything kids can bang together to make lots of noise is sheer delight to them. Muffin pans, foil pie plates, plastic margarine tubs, and old Tupperware containers and lids will give your child a fine head start as a professional Frisbee Golfer.

*W*hen Meredith was a toddler, I'd put small cans and boxes in the lower cupboards so she could "grocery-shop" while I was busy making dinner or whatever. Sometimes I'd have to search the whole house to find that can of sliced mushrooms I knew I'd bought, but on the positive side, long before she was school-age, Meredith had learned all the letters of the alphabet, and even quite a few words, from looking at the labels on those cans and boxes. I can guarantee you she was the first kid in class who knew how to spell "linguine."

Caroline
piano teacher

Keep a bin in the kitchen and the family room to hold some of your child's toys. It will make her feel that her activities have meaning, and that her things have a place in this communal space, along with the rest of the family's. If you keep a stack of your magazines and books on the coffee table, let her keep her own small stack of reading material there too.

Let your child be a part of special family dinners and put down a plastic "splat mat" in your dining room rather than relegating the little guy to the kids table. If your dining-room chairs are upholstered in fabric, you can protect them by using removable, clear plastic seat covers on the children's chairs. When you entertain grown-ups, just remove the covers. Unless you happen to hang out with a lot of slobs.

Another way to make your house kid-friendly is through decoration. If you're one of those women who had her pre-kid house oh-so-carefully decorated in Minimalist Asian or English Country, get over your tasteful self, because your new style's about to become Toddler Traditional. The trick is, don't fight it—work with it. That big, inflatable Valentine's heart that you couldn't resist getting your crawdler at the carnival becomes a shabby-chic icon if it's put together with similar funky furnishings. In fact, you may find yourself not missing that raw-silk shoji screen after all. And if you do, well, just put it away with the rugs and the coffee table and bring it out when they're so embarrassed by you that they don't want to be in the house anymore.

MORE OTHER MOTHERS' TIPS

- Never let a crawdler go barefoot in public (no-brainer).
- Keep dog and cat food out of your child's reach.
- Flea bites and pet germs can be dangerous to humans; keep your dog or cat clean and healthy.
- Keep your kitty litter boxes away from your kiddies.
- Send your dog through obedience training, preferably before the baby arrives.
- Crawdlers can get trapped under your bed; either raise it or lower it.
- Crawdlers can also get trapped under the leg-rest of a recliner; make sure yours is safe.
- No strings, tags, ribbons, ties, etc., on a crawdler's clothing; they can and will get tangled in everything.
- Buy carpets and upholstery with patterns; they won't show dirt or stains like solid-color furnishings will.
- Share a babysitter with another mom so that you can leave your kids at home while you go shopping.

IT'S IN THE BAG

When your child becomes mobile, the following items should be with you at all times:

- Disposable diapers
- Baby wipes
- Juice
- Sippy cup
- Jar of baby food
- Spoon and fork
- Bibs
- Cheerios
- Toys
- Ziploc baggies
- Packet of tissues
- Cell phone, with your pediatrician's number and 911 on speed dial
- Wallet
- Keys
- Hairbrush
- Cosmetics bag
- Band-Aid "Plus" bandages with antibiotics

4

"Cry Like a Baby"

(What <u>You'll</u> Be Doing When Your Child Hits the Terrible Twos)

The phrase "terrible twos" is a complete misnomer. Toddlers don't enter that stage at two but much earlier, around fourteen to eighteen months. And it doesn't always end automatically when they turn three, either; sometimes it goes on until they're middle-aged.

From the moment your child is born, your mission is to form a fully functioning, capable, responsible, independent adult—and, God willing, one who can support you in your old age, because you'll be bankrupt from paying for college. This is why the terrible-twos stage exists: to help toddlers learn to assert themselves as individuals, with their own will and consciousness; and, Mom and Dad, to teach you that your child is a separate being (they cut the cord in the delivery room, remember?).

L... two years: she's
learne... k, talk, feed herself, a... like Band-Aids.
Almos... closer to estab-
lishing... ccept; others are
awed a... a few hard-won
words

Bu...

This Is

The fir... chasing after a
crawdle... picking up after
a dropp... a treat. Unless
the kid's... Here's how the
game is

Put... s at least a foot
or two o... ve seconds, he
will have... e floor. Do all
toddlers... gravity? Partly.
But they... hat goes on in
their ado... his: "Mommy
always do... out it, there's
probably... it be I'm the
boss of h... drop this and
watch Mo... aaaaay!!!!"

Our first instinct is to pick up the toy, clean it off, and hand it back to the kid. But after you've done this fifty or sixty times it starts getting a little old.

What the Other Mothers Know

Put the baby on the floor! If he's on the floor, then *he* can pick up whatever he drops.

There, that was easy, wasn't it?

(This tip courtesy of Mrs. Sir Isaac Newton.)

When they drop something out of the high chair, pick it up and hand it back to them. But if they drop it again, you know that they're trying to test you. So, each time it happens, add a minute to the length of time it takes you to return the object to them. It doesn't take long before they realize that this game is going to get more and more boring if they keep it up.

Another tip is, don't let discipline turn into a labor-management dispute. The first time you tell Junior not to shove pieces of hot dog into the air-conditioning vent, you patiently explain that we don't do that (don't bother to explain BTUs and compressors, since even adults can't understand that anyway). When your little recidivist does it again, you take the hot dog away. Once it's clear that they're deliberately being oppositional, take action; don't discuss it or try to reason with them. They *know* they're not supposed to be doing it; that's *why* they're doing it.

Sometimes it helps to give terrible two-ers something that they're legitimately allowed to be assertive over—like telling Rover to sit. It probably won't accomplish anything in terms of training your pet but it temporarily makes kids feel like they're in charge of something. And it'll keep them out of your hair for a good ten minutes—until they realize it's more fun trying to boss Mom than it is the dog.

What Part of "No" Don't You Understand?

The first time your child says "no" to you rather than obediently do what she's told will take you aback, that's for sure. But not all "no"s are necessarily accompanied by a full-blown temper tantrum, either.

*O*ne day, when Rena was not yet two, she discovered how to lean against her open bedroom door, bump her butt into it, and make it slam shut. I told her, "Don't do that, Rena, you might pinch yourself." She did it again. And again I told her, "No." Then she did it a third time. I looked at her and said, "No!" She drew herself up, put her hands on her hips, and said, very sternly, "Mommy, don't you say 'no' to me!" I am very proud of myself that I didn't do the first two things that came to mind. One was, burst out laughing, because there I was, six feet tall, squaring off against a twenty-two-month-old who barely came up to my shin. The second thing was to say, "Go in your room and shut up." What I did was tell myself, *Take a deep breath,* and then I said, aloud, "Rena, when you're doing something that could hurt you, I *will* say 'no' to you, and you *will* listen." Of course, that's when she was tiny. Now she's six. At this point, I'd say, "Go in your room and shut up."

Margaret
city planner

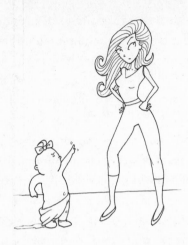

What the Other Mothers Know

Laugh *with* a child, never *at*. Here's an example of how tough it is not to laugh when a kid ventures an insult: one day, after Michele disciplined her four-year-old Marc for some infraction, he furrowed his little brow and, in a desperate attempt to summon the sharpest, most humiliating, most devastating insult he could, spat out, "Your jokes aren't funny!" (She's laughing just writing that sentence.)

But, there's nothing in the Official Mom Rulebook that says you can't chortle quietly. Come on, how can you not giggle at thirty pounds of apple-juice breath and poopy pants standing up to an adult? How can you not marvel at her newfound independence? But most of all, how can you make sure she never does it again?

As soon as you finish yocking it up inwardly, wipe that smile off your face and replace it with one of quiet and serious determination, because, ladies, what we're talking about here is nothing less than the eternal struggle between the forces of Order and the forces of Darkness. It is a struggle you can, and must, always win. The secret to winning? Never let your child become aware that it's a struggle, and never let her think that it's winnable by anyone but Mom and Dad.

One of the keys to this is never taking your child's actions personally. Little kids will, generally, express two kinds of negative (over)reactions. The first occurs when they're told to do something they don't want to do—like finishing their puréed zucchini (ugh, can you blame them?) or turning off the TV. The second kind of negative reaction occurs when they realize that *you're* not going to do everything *they* want you to do. The results can be so difficult, so trying, that it seems like every other day you're ready to beg your doctor to put you on a Stoli drip.

This is where learning to *choose your battles* comes in. You can't tell two- and three-year-olds "no" all the time, because if you said "no" to everything you don't want them to do, you'll never say anything other than "no" all day long. Therefore, you must pick and choose your "no"s (as opposed to picking and choosing your nose). When it comes to the important battles—things related to safety, health, socialization, and intellectual development—"no" is a complete sentence. But some of those things you're fighting over probably aren't so vital.

*W*hen my daughter Amy was around three, she decided there was no reason why socks had to match. Why should she choose between wearing her green Kermit the Frog socks and her Hello Kitty socks, when she could wear one of each? I tried to explain that it looked kind of funny, but the more insistent I became, the more resistant she was. As I heard my voice growing louder and louder, I suddenly thought, *What difference does it make? Either the kids'll tease her, or she'll start a fad.* So, she went to a birthday party with mismatched socks, the other kids told her it looked kind of funny, and she never did it again.

Halley
real-estate developer

Does it really matter if your little boy insists on stacking his plastic rings with the little ones on the bottom? If it's not that important, just say "yes."

Temper, Temper

The first time your child throws a bona fide temper tantrum is a gob-smacking shocker. Here is your angelic, sweet, cuddly, loving little babe suddenly turning purple with rage, screaming like a pint-size Donald Trump minus the comb-over, gulping air so deeply to keep his mad on that he literally sucks all the oxygen out of the room, like a reverse hurricane.

You and your husband stare at one another with eyes big as hubcaps from disbelief.

"Where did that come from?"

"I don't know, but is it too late to change his name to Damien?"

What the Other Mothers Know

Again, never give in to that impulse to laugh. It will only make your child angrier, and delay you from getting to the root of the problem and dealing with it. And never, ever lose your temper. All you'll do is frighten your child, set a bad example, and ruin your mascara.

*T*he first time Maria ever threw a temper tantrum, it caught me totally by surprise. I had put her into her play yard so I could do some laundry. She loved her play yard and it was a large space, so it wasn't like she was being penned in or anything; and all her favorite toys were in there. I think it had to do with the fact that she didn't like me moving her, like she wanted to be her own boss? Well, she started shrieking, "No! No! Out!" When I just stood there, looking at her in shock, she threw herself down on the floor—thank God for carpeting—and started beating her fists on it! So, I instinctively did what I'd seen my own mom do with my younger sisters and brother. I shrugged at her and said, "Fine, throw yourself down." I didn't react. I refused to let myself get freaked out by it. She started screaming louder. So I said, "We'll just wait till you're done," and then I went off to put in a load of wash. When I came back ten minutes later, she was happy as a clam, playing with her blocks.

Suzanne
homemaker

When a child has a tantrum, it's best to pay as little attention to her as possible. So long as she's in a physically safe location where she can't throw anything or hurt herself or someone else, let her stay there to cool off. Speak calmly and firmly, and stay in control of yourself. Give her no attention until she begins to calm down. When she does, give her positive, calm approval for it.

Another way of getting the tantrummer to cease and desist is simply to move him into another part of the house. Not the cellar or a closet, for Pete's sake, but the dining room, or the living room—somewhere you can see them.

A friend once asked me what to do to keep from beating the crap out of your three-year-old, and I told her that what you do is lock yourself in the bathroom and cry. Then, as your crying subsides, you'll hear someone outside the door, crying, too (either from making Mommy cry or because you won't let him into the bathroom). At that point, you open the door and give him a big hug, then you cry together. Of course, most of them understand perfectly if you say, "Mommy needs a time out" and go off by yourself for a few minutes.

Paula
graduate student

Usually a tiny terror is so shocked to see Mommy weep (obviously he's never watched Mommy weigh herself) or give herself a time out that it stops him dead in his tantrumming tracks, turning him from a participant into an observer. "Huh? *She's* supposed to be the adult in this relationship, she's not supposed to act like me!" Does it make them realize how ridiculous someone looks throwing a fit? Who knows? Used sparingly, it's a very effective way of getting them to stop the inappropriate behavior long enough for you to inject some calm and reason into the situation, before you turn into Momzilla.

Pick Up or Shut Up

Children, like all humans no matter their age, despise rules yet long for them at the same time. Maybe we just like having rules so we can enjoy breaking them. But we all have to have them, and even though little kids rebel against them like crazy, they need them more than anyone else.

Among the first rules a child learns is putting away his toys. After that, it's going down for bed and naps; then eating the proper foods; then not testing his brand-new baby sister's fontanel with a ball-peen hammer. But it's the toys that comprise the first big discipline area for kids.

In chapter 2, we already gave you several tips for conning little ones into helping pick up their toys by making a game out of it; but what do you do when they're too old to be conned and still too young to understand a bribe?

What the Other Mothers Know

Jennifer was three when I started asking her to put away her toys. She'd pick up one or two, then she'd either get distracted or launch into a fit of protracted whining. So I bought some large plastic bins and put them in her room and the family room. That night, I told her the red bin was for dolls, the blue bin was for stuffed animals, and the yellow bin was for toys. Anything she didn't put away would go into the *green* bin, and nothing in there could come out again until the red, blue, and yellow bins were full. She picked up some of her toys that night. The next morning, she wanted to play with a toy I'd placed in the green bin, and she threw a fit when I wouldn't let her. That afternoon, when it came time to pick up her other toys, she did; and next morning, all the toys from the green bin were "paroled." Once was all it took to teach her that what comes out must be put away.

Laura
charitable-foundation director

Don't worry that this might not work with your child because he has a giga-lection of toys to choose from. All it takes sometimes is just a "no" from Mom to suddenly turn a so-so toy into Toy Number One, and make him just have to have it.

An English friend of ours used to talk to her toddler about his toys in a very particular way:

I believe I first heard this expression from my grandmother, who, whenever I'd help dry the dinner dishes, would ask me to put the glass or plate back "where it lives." So when my little boy, Geoffrey, was old enough to start picking up after himself, I remembered Grandmum and said, "Time to put away your toys, Geoffrey. And where does Mr. Potato Head live?" By anthropomorphizing these inanimate objects, I got him to respect his toys and to feel more responsible for putting them away. Of course, I did once have to retrieve a Beanie Baby from the potty after Geoffrey decided it needed to learn how to swim.

Anne

landscape architect

Unfortunately, these techniques won't work on older kids. If you tried to pull the holding-bin gambit on a twelve- or thirteen-year-old with the stuff he just drops on the floor, his room would be completely empty: cell phone, clothes, laptop, CDs, video games, DVDs, books (yes, some kids actually still read), backpack—you'd have to throw out every single thing he owned. And don't even bother trying to convince him his iPod has feelings.

A-one and A-two . . .

When your child reaches the age of four or so, and has begun to learn numbers, you can start the NASA Countdown Warning Method of discipline. Let's say you've told your sweet little fellow that it's time to turn off the TV and take his nap, and he starts screaming like coach Bobby Knight during March Madness . . .

I always hated hearing any parent give the warning countdown. "All right, I'm going to count to five, and . . ." It sounded so old-fashioned and bossy; just tell the kid what to do. Then one day, when Samantha was four, she and I were at a friend's house, and she was playing in the pool with my friend's six-year-old. At noon, my friend said, "It's time for lunch, kids, let's get out of the pool." She stood there by the steps, but they ignored her and kept on playing. Then she lowered her voice and said, "Okay, I'm going to count to five." Before she even got to "two," her daughter had grabbed Sam and pulled her out of the pool as if she'd suddenly noticed a shark in there.

Dee
museum curator

What the Other Mothers Know

Kids might not always like limits, but they want them. And you don't even necessarily have to get all the way up to "five," either; just start counting. Even if the kid's three years old and has no idea what numbers mean, it's the tone of voice and the look you give them that convey the message, "No fooling around, pal; this is for real."

After Dee started using the countdown method to great success, she found herself in the produce section of her grocery store one day, where she began counting out how many apples she needed for a pie she was going to make. Suddenly she noticed Samantha staring at the apples and shaking her head.

"What's the matter, Sam?"

"Those poor little apples don't know how much trouble they're in."

But He's Such an Angel at Home!

It's one thing to handle a child's temper tantrum at home, and another thing altogether if he has a tantrum in public. For starters, it's embarrassing when your child acts out in front of others, for the simple reason that it makes you think that anyone witnessing the tantrum must think your child is the devil incarnate and you are a bad mother. (Of course, your child is only mildly possessed, and you're a perfect mom.) But don't sweat it; most of the time people aren't really thinking that anyway.

*M*y husband and I were attending his law firm's picnic with our three-year-old son, Josh. While my husband was off playing softball, Josh saw the older kids picking sides for a softball game of their own and wanted to join in; obviously, I wouldn't let him, because they would've ended up using him for second base. Before I could stop him, he ran over to the equipment and picked up a bat. I took it from him and he started to howl. An older man, who was dressed like he was the janitor or something, very kindly told me that Josh's reaction indicated I had a future ballplayer on my hands. He said he remembered how hard it is for little kids to stand aside and watch the big ones have all the fun, so he played catch with Josh. After fifteen minutes, Josh conked out on a picnic blanket. Later, I found out that the "janitor" was one of the firm's senior partners. Every year he sees Josh at the picnic and asks him how his game is coming along. And this season, when Josh's Little League team needed a sponsor, guess who came to the rescue? Yes, my eight-year-old pitcher is a Finley, Gold-stein, Perelskin Pirate.

Heather
portrait artist

What the Other Mothers Know

There's nothing wrong with getting a little help calming down a fussing child. Sometimes all they need is a little diversion from the temptations at hand to get "right" again. If the situation absolutely compels you to discipline your child in front of other adults and they give you the stink eye, just ignore it. Or you can do what our friend Joanne did:

*O*ne afternoon I took Maggie, then two years old, to our local park. We were having a great time until she decided she *had* to go on the slide. I'd recently had knee surgery, and climbing up a slide was not going to be in my exercise program for a while, so I said no. She threw a fit. Full-blown, that kind where it looks like they're going to burst a blood vessel? Several other moms started to stare, giving me a look like, *God, you have a spoiled brat.* So I thought, what the hell, and went over to one who had an older child. Trying to make myself heard above Maggie's thousand-decibel screams, I asked her if she had any pointers for a mom new to the terrible twos. Well, like almost all people when you ask for advice, she was flattered and immediately warmed up. She suggested I take Maggie into the car, put her in the car seat, and wait silently for her to ride it out. Always keep a magazine or a book handy, she said, because a time-out can give a mom a chance to catch up on back issues of magazines. It took nearly fifteen minutes, but finally Maggie recovered. And during that time I actually managed to read *Newsweek*. There was something about a hurricane Katrina that had hit New Orleans; who knew?

Joanne
homemaker

Always ask the Other Mothers for guidance, even if you don't know them personally. Most people enjoy sharing their expertise. For one thing, it makes them feel good to help others. For another, it gives them an opportunity to show off what they know to someone who's actually listening, for a change.

Different Folks for Different Strokes

There will be times when you're not only taking care of your terrible-two-er, but someone else's as well. (Could this be called a terrible-two-fer?) If your wee guest starts to throw a fit at your place, on your watch, what do you do? And how do you know if your method of discipline is the same as the other mother's? And whether that mom, hearing that you've disciplined her child, won't claw your eyes out?

What the Other Mothers Know

When you're responsible for watching someone else's child in your home, your rules rule. This is vital not only for your sanity but to reinforce in your own child that the rules of the house are to be followed by one and all.

*A*s far as behavior goes, whenever another child is in my house or coming with me someplace, I'm the boss and there's no doubt about it. I'm the alpha dog (or perhaps I should say alpha bitch). Recently I had an old friend from out of town visiting with her four-year-old son. We were both standing there when he reached down and deliberately yanked my dog's tail, and I corrected him very strongly. And then I thought, *Uh-oh.* I looked over at my friend, but before I could stammer an apology, she gratefully said, "Please, keep doing it!"

Cheryl

attorney

When you leave your child in a friend's care, make sure your friend knows that as far as you're concerned, she's in charge. So long as there's no doubt in your mind that your friend will do the right thing, trust her discipline, if it's necessary.

There are also times when we are with our child in someone else's home—and they don't share out parenting ideals. This can be tricky.

I have a friend who has three boys, ages three to eight, and the house is totally wild. I'm a pretty relaxed mother but she makes me look like I'm the most uptight human being on earth. You go over there and it is chaos—the first twenty minutes we're there, my daughter Sarah, who's three and a half, doesn't quite know what to make of it, so she'll hang on to my leg. Then she gets acclimated and she's off like a rocket; she loves running with the boys. My friend also allows them to eat in front of the television. It makes my skin crawl, but they're really good parents and the kids are happy and polite. And Sarah has the greatest time.

Afterwards, though, at home, all I hear is, "But I get to do that at Tommy's house." And I say, "That's Tommy's house. There are things you do at Tommy's house that you cannot do in our house. Everybody's house is different." I don't think she quite got the concept, so, the next time I had to run errands I took her with me. I made the point that we can't buy ice cream at the dry cleaners, or pick up our clothes from the grocery store. They're all stores, but each is different, just like every house is different. I think she sort of understood, but whenever we get an invitation to Tommy's house, she's thrilled.

Theresa
teacher

Your little one needs to understand—and will, eventually—that different rules apply to different settings. In some houses, he's allowed to read at the dinner table; in other houses, he isn't. At school, he's not allowed to swing on his stomach, because the teacher can't watch him every single second, but if he's with you or Dad at the park, it's okay, because he's never out of your sight. And you don't have thirty-two other kids to watch.

You have to adapt when you're a guest in someone else's home, and you must prepare your child for that as well. "We're going to so-and-so's house. Because it's their house, we have to do what that mommy says. And even though we let you jump on the sofa in our house, that other mommy might *not* think it's okay to jump on her sofas. In different houses, different rules apply."

And if none of these tips works out that well, just think of it as teaching your kid social Darwinism: adapt, or you'll go the way of the dinosaurs.

Sit Down with Your Sitter

We spoke in chapter 3 about child care, and about hiring help in your home. When your child enters the terrible twos, sit down with your nanny or babysitter or housekeeper and lay out some ground rules for behavior and discipline. Crime and punishment should be consistent from parent to employee, or the child will get mixed signals. Teach your child to show respect to everyone, and above all, that includes employees in your home: a housekeeper or nanny is a stand-in for Mom and Dad. If it's any comfort, though, terrible two-ers tend to save their worst possible behavior for their parents, not the "help." Probably because it's just not as much fun tormenting folks who get to leave at five o'clock.

What the Other Mothers Know

Don't allow your children to take advantage of the situation.

*M*y husband and I have friends we love dearly, but the way they speak to their housekeeper is terribly curt and brusque. Of course, their child now speaks to this woman the same way. What they do in their own home is their business, but I noticed that after my three-year-old had been there for a play date, she spoke to our housekeeper, Mercedes, the same way. I almost took her head off. I said, "You do not tell Mercedes to do anything. You ask her, 'please, would you,' or 'please, may I.' And most of all, you always say 'thank you'!" The next time our friends' daughter came here to play, I heard her speak rudely to Mercedes. I marched in there and read her the riot act too. Now the little girl is more polite to her housekeeper than her parents are. I guess that's a little progress.

Arlene

homemaker

Don't allow your child to think she can get away with riding rough-shod over a housekeeper or a nanny. And above all, don't create an atmosphere in your home where your child's caregiver will feel uncomfortable or afraid to tell you how your child is behaving. Reassure her that you want her to be honest.

It's All Going to Pot

The two words besides "terrible twos" that strike even more terror into the hearts of parents are: "potty" and "training."

Your child will forge her independence from you in two primary ways.

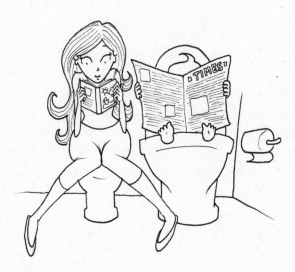

The first is from the mouth end, screaming at you in a tantrum. The second is from the *other* end.

There probably have been more books written about potty-training than any other aspect of early child-rearing. It can go smooth as silk, or it can be a prolonged and protracted battle that goes on for a year. We all live for the day when we don't have to change another dirty diaper; and for working moms who have to place their children into nursery school or preschool day care, potty-training is especially important, because some schools or centers won't take kids unless they're house-broken.

What the Other Mothers Know

What follow are some of the smartest, savviest, most devious and successful courses of potty-training we know of. Read and learn.

*M*y daughter Emily had accident after accident. It took so long and was such a bother that I resisted training Jack for a long time. He was in Pull-Ups before he could walk, because he was too big for regular disposables to really fit, so I knew I couldn't use them as a training tool. Well, here's how I potty-trained him (drum roll, please): I waited for him to beg me to let him use the potty.

Whenever we'd go out to eat, Emily would invariably wait until we'd just been served and then announce that she had to go potty. So, one night we were out and Jack said he needed to go too. I said, "No, Jack, you can't use the potty." After several instances of this, and Jack getting more and more upset,

I said, "You have to use the potty five times at home before you can use the potty in a restaurant." I rewarded him for going in the potty by letting him go in a potty! It worked, though; I couldn't believe how fast he was trained.

Doriana

veterinarian

Maureen gets the Academy Award for Best Actress in a Potty-training Role:

*H*enry wouldn't even look at the potty. At three and a half, he was still crying, "I love my diapie!"

My husband's mom had mailed him a box of things from his child-hood, and in it was a pair of rubber pants, the kind toddlers used to wear over cloth diapers. But these were thirty years old, so the rubber was all cracked and yellowed (why she saved them and sent them I don't know, but that's a whole other issue). Henry was really into Buzz Lightyear, so I bought him a bunch of Buzz underpants. When he woke up the next morning, I took off his diaper and said, "You have three choices. You can go around with no diaper, and no pants, which might be embarrassing at the park. Or you can wear Daddy's old underwear. Or you can wear Buzz." He saw those old rubber pants and practically gagged. "No, don't make me wear those!" he said. "I pick Buzz!" So he wore his Buzz Light-year underpants and stayed dry as a bone for two hours until he sat down on the potty, all by himself, and went. He hasn't had one accident.

Maureen

journalist

Our friend Kerry decided to go for a time-honored method when her daughter, Melissa, was three years and two months old:

We'd tried training Melissa for weeks and weeks and nothing seemed to work. I'd read two books, hit potty-training Web sites, bought the bells-and-whistles potty—all of it. Everything I read said to avoid giving tangible rewards for going in the potty, and everyone said the worst reward you could give them was candy. Well, after weeks and weeks of going through this and failing, one day I got an idea. I told her that if she took off her diaper by herself and sat down on the potty, she'd get part of her treat. That sort of intrigued her. Treat . . . ? So she sat down all full of curiosity, while I went into the kitchen and scooped out half a dish of chocolate ice cream. Melissa is a born chocolate hound, so I knew this would get her attention. I brought it back to the bathroom and gave it to her. Yes, I know it sounds sort of gross, eating in the bathroom, but a mom's gotta do what a mom's gotta do. So I said, "When you're done going pee-pee in the potty, you can have the other half of the scoop." I had no sooner walked out the door than I heard that distinctive trickle, followed by a proud "All done, Mommy." That was it. The kid's a female; what greater inducement is there in life for us women than chocolate?

Kerry
illustrator

But after you've trained your child, don't get flush with your success.

$\mathcal{D}$ana potty-trained very easily at two years and eight months, and by the time she turned three, she hadn't had one accident. We live in an apartment complex with a pool; one day in August, while I was at work, my husband took her swimming, and guess who pooped in the pool? Hint: it was not my husband. The pool had to be shut down for a week; and, after word got out who was responsible, my husband and I had to suffer these hostile looks every time we ran into someone in the halls or the mail room. Of course, since I'm the mom, the nastiest looks were reserved for *me*. So, we learned our lesson: you never set foot outside the apartment without putting her on the potty first, even if she says she doesn't have to go.

Joyce
teacher

Joyce also made sure her husband understood that if he ever again forgot to take Dana to the bathroom before swimming, he'd be the one who'd have to dive in with the net.

Potty-training is even more problematic at night; we all like to get our eight hours, but we don't want to change sopping-wet sheets the next morning, either. Here's a tip from Ilene: wake up your child at ten p.m., take him to the potty, then put him back to bed immediately. Do this for three nights in a row, then move the wake-up time to ten *fifteen* p.m. Again, do this for three nights in a row, and keep adding fifteen minutes every few days until you reach midnight. The later in the evening that the child uses the potty, the longer he'll stay dry, eventually making it all the way through to morning. Of course, this is predicated on either you or your husband being a night owl who can stay up until twelve; if neither of you is, then alternate nights. Or try to think of a way you can keep each other up till midnight. Just be careful, or you'll wind up with another bed-wetter in nine months.

And take advantage of waterproof mattress protectors.

Clothes Make the Kid

Another battleground during the terrible twos is teaching kids how to dress themselves. Making it into a game is always a good idea.

What the Other Mothers Know

One thing I teach my preschool kids—and now my grandson, Brandon— is how to put on their own coats. Brandon puts his coat on the floor in front of his feet, with the inside showing and the hood (or the label, if there is no hood) closest to his feet. He bends over, puts his arms in the sleeves, and flips the coat over his head. All that's left to do is to zip the coat. Believe me, getting ten three-year-olds ready to go outside is a lot easier when they can help themselves. And they're very proud.

Trisha
preschool teacher

You might also try the Legend of the Ghost Pajamas:

*T*rying to get my four-year-old son into pajamas at night was like trying to rope a buttered calf. But he always loved scary bedtime stories. So, one night, in desperation, I made up the Legend of the Ghost Pajamas. I held up his pajama top and bottoms and made them dance around the room as if they were being worn by an invisible kid ghost, all the while making spooky "woooooooo" noises. I told Todd that the ghost pajamas could only be defeated if he put them on. He scrambled to get them over his chubby little legs and arms, and as he did, I made these gasping, choking sounds as the ghost was vanquished. It never failed: night after night, Todd defeated the ghost pajamas and I got to sleep a half-hour earlier. Now he's off at college, where he's probably playing a different kind of pajama game.

Carla
Homemaker

But the problem isn't always *how* to get them dressed, it's the *what*. This is when your child refuses to wear a particular outfit, or, as happened to our friend below, will wear only one outfit.

*F*or two or three months, when Jasmine was four years old, she wore a tank top we called her "rainbow shirt" *all the time*. It was a constant struggle to get her to wear anything else, and it was especially worrisome, because it was winter. Then my friend Debbie had an idea and came over with her Polaroid camera. She had Jasmine try on everything in her closet and photographed her in each outfit, making a game of it. When Jasmine saw the pictures and realized how cute she looked in all the other cloth-ing, she was willing to let me throw her rainbow shirt into the laundry and put on something else. I taped Debbie's photos inside the door of Jasmine's closet. Now she's ten years old, and I only wish she was happy with just one outfit; her clothing bills are putting me into debt.

Grace
architect

This was a great solution to a real problem, one that was especially critical in the morning, when Grace was trying to get Jasmine ready for school and get herself to work on time. Unless a school uniform is required, don't let clothes be too much of a priority. Again, you must always choose your battles.

Excuse Me, <u>What</u> Did You Say?!

The final "frontier" of the terrible twos/threes/fours is related to the potty but not in the way you think. It's teaching your kid not to have a potty *mouth*.

*O*ne day at the park, when Michael was three years old, there were kids a few years older than him, who used really bad language. In the maybe ten minutes he was within earshot of those kids, he picked up the F-word and "a**hole." That night, my husband said, "You know, Michael, you need to go sit down," and Mikey goes, "You know, Dad, you're a f***ing a**hole." Three years old! My husband and I talked with him about it and told him that certain people use certain words and those aren't the kind of words he needs to use. Michael sat there and he listened and nodded the whole time and then he goes, "Daddy, I'm really sorry I called you a f***ing a**hole." We stopped frequenting that particular park.

Sasha

photographer

What the Other Mothers Know

Linguistically, little kids are sponges. They hear a word once and they can repeat it. Often, they can repeat it at the most embarrassing times and in the most inappropriate places. And if they can see on your face that a particular dirty word has hit its mark, they'll keep on using it until you tell them not to.

Make it abundantly clear to them that there are simply some things that grown-ups are allowed to say and do that kids are not allowed to say and do. No, it isn't fair, but that's just the way it is. It often helps to point out that *Mommy* can't use certain words at certain times and places either. We don't think this is a circumstance when you reason with them. Warn them that if they use the word again, they lose a privilege, or a toy.

And if that advice doesn't work for your kid, resist the urge to try a bar of soap. Or, better yet, isolate them from other kids, for a nice, healthy time-out. But close the door tight, in case he starts swearing like a high-pitched sailor on shore leave.

While we're on the subject of language, there's the issue of nomenclature. Specifically, what language do you want your child to use when referring to his or her bodily parts and functions?

Some parents insist on teaching their child the clinical, technical, Greco-Latin terms: defecate, urinate, vagina, penis, etc. Others are happy referring to buttocks as hiney, fanny, tushie, and so on. We honestly don't know how you teach a three-year-old to refer to gas as flatulence, but maybe there are some really smart kids who can pronounce that word.

Then there's that third tier of words that are acceptable to an adult but may be a little too crude for kids: words like "fart" and "wiener." (How could you even teach a kid those words and keep a straight face?) And then there are those little-kid words that most parents use only around the house: poo-poo, doody, wee-wee, etc. Little kids are comfortable using those words at home, but when they use them at school, they're either likely to be told the clinical terms by a teacher, or risk being laughed at by the other kids for using baby words. And what two-and-half-year-old would understand the expression "I gotta go see a man about a dog"?

When Abby was three and in nursery school, she came home giggling about so-and-so having "farted" at nap time. My husband and I felt that word was a shade too crude until she was at least Nickelodeon age, so we wracked our brains to come up with a word that meant "fart" but that wasn't as explicit as "passing gas," as clinical as "flatulence," or as old-fashioned as "breaking wind." Then, a word just popped into my head: "zorch." It sounded vaguely flatulent, but not onomatopoeic; and it didn't sound baby-ish. So, that's what our family has stuck with for the past sixteen years, employed both as a noun and a verb. Feel free to use "zorch" if you like, with your own child, or better yet, make up a phrase of your own.

Michele

Let's be honest here: the persons your child is most likely to hear dirty words from are you and your husband. Ilene remembers an incident when her daughter was two and a half; Nikka, who was in her high chair, dropped a cookie on the floor and fired off the S-word in frustration. Knowing full well that she had learned this word from them, Ilene and her husband decided that their home was henceforth a "language-free zone."

There are, of course, those special moments when no amount of self-discipline can prevent a parent from uttering a four-letter word—such as when she opens the mail and discovers that the IRS is auditing her tax returns going back to 1989. What some parents do when this occurs is pay a fine by depositing a dollar into what we like to call a Cussin' Kitty. After $10 has accumulated, let your child use it toward buying a book or toy he's had his eye on.

If your child persists in using foul language, turn the tables and fine *him* fifty cents each time you hear him utter a nasty—or, depending on how fat his piggy bank is, a whole dollar. And make him watch while you remove the money; seeing the bill disappear into Mom's wallet is a lot more sobering to a kid than being told after the fact.

These are tough years, the twos and threes. But guess what? As the age-old cross-cultural adage goes, "Little children, little problems. Big children, big problems." Yes, even more challenging issues are yet to come. So, use this stage to really learn how to parent: to be consistent, fair, and dependable. It's the best way to lay the groundwork for your children to feel safe about coming to you with whatever big problems may arise.

And as for your mini-monster, we promise you, things start to improve when children are around four. Hanging out with their contemporaries teaches them that while tantrums sometimes work on adults, don't try 'em on other kids. There's nothing like the scorn of one's peers to cure tantrum-itis.

MORE OTHER MOTHERS' TIPS

- Set aside a specific space for your child to chill if he has a tantrum, like the floor of his bedroom, or a corner of the family room.
- Clear a space for *you* for when your child has a tantrum (laundry rooms are good—you can wait out the storm *and* do a load of wash).
- If you absolutely have to take your child into a temptations-heavy store, put her in a shopping cart so she can't reach for toys and candy on the shelves.
- Keep children's books near the potty.
- Keep grown-up reading material by the big potty so you can accompany your child while he or she sits on the "mini-throne."
- Keep Ziplocs or plastic grocery bags at the bottom of the clothes hamper for separating wet or soiled underpants; keep them in your car, too.

IT'S IN THE BAG

- Baby wipes (just in case)
- Change of undies if trained, diapers if not
- Lose the pacifier already!
- Sippy cup
- Ziplocs (so much for this no longer being a diaper bag)
- One toy
- Cheerios
- Fat Crayolas (for chubby hands)
- Simple coloring-book pages
- Bib with trough
- Portable splat mats
- Change of clothing
- Sunscreen
- Cell phone, with psychiatrist's number on speed dial
- Wallet
- A book or magazine for you
- CDs to listen to in the car
- Blankie
- Gin in a childproof container
- Cat-o'-nine-tails
- Small-size perfume and cosmetics samples because it's mighty crowded in there

5

"I Found a Million-dollar Baby"

(And That's What It'll Cost to Put Him Through Nursery School)

Raising a child is a demanding job, whether you do it part-time or full-time, and everybody needs support. Imagine if you're new to the area, know few people, maybe don't work, and then you have a baby. That's where a Mommy and Me class could be a real lifesaver. Not that learning the Hokey Pokey is going to get your kid into Yale, but taking one of those classes can introduce you to an entire network of Other Mothers.

What the Other Mothers Know

Mommy and Me, Gymboree, and My Gym classes take babies even as young as "0 months old." We don't know what 0 months really means—

still in utero?—but there's a class for 'em if you want one. Such classes are offered virtually all over the country, from the biggest city to the tiniest hamlet, at fairly reasonable prices.

Of course, you might ask exactly how much socializing can a newborn do, other than follow Mom with his eyes; and he can't even do that until he's a few weeks old. It's one thing to schlep a three-month-old who looks like a live bobblehead doll to stare and drool at other three-month-olds, but it's another thing entirely for a crawling, sitting up, bright-eyed six-month-old who's getting his first glimpse of other six-month-olds. If your kid's a stay-at-home, whether he's being cared for by you or by a nanny, by eighteen months he will need the company of other children.

If you can't find a Gymboree, Mommy and Me, My Gym, or other commercial playgroup in your area, check for a private playgroup at your church or temple; local public library; the community calendar section of your newspaper; local college; and the Internet. If there are no other moms of young children on your block, start looking for them at the park, at the grocery store, anywhere you can find them.

And if that yields no results, you can always do what Audrey did and start your own playgroup.

My husband and I were still in school when our son was born, and money was so tight that I decided to see if I could find some parents and start our own playgroup. I posted flyers at our local market, our pediatrician's office, the student union, and a children's clothing store. After I received e-mails from three likely-sounding parents, we decided to get together for coffee one Saturday morning and see how we got along. We discussed types of activities, what days and times to meet, snack assignments, and how to rotate hosting on a weekly basis. We are and remain a mixed group: one is an African-American registered nurse; another is a voice coach; and our fourth "mom" is a gay stay-at-home dad. Our babies are now in first grade and attending different schools but we still hang out together—though sometimes it's around a poker table.

Audrey
dietician

Every mother we spoke to who'd taken such classes felt that their main value was to introduce moms to other moms, and we all know of lifelong friendships that were forged in playgroups when the kids were itty-bitties. In other words, they're designed less for Me than they are for Mommy, especially first-time mommies.

If you don't like the other moms in your playgroup, find another one.

Lake Forest is a very wealthy suburb of Chicago, but not everybody who lives here is rich. When Jason was eight months old, we joined a Mommy and Me class that met weekly. Most of the babies were very sweet, and at that age, how can they not get along? Except about half of this group was Housekeeper and Me. And as for the moms who did show up, I didn't expect to be sitting in a circle with mostly first-time moms discussing such "mommy" things as their new tennis court, or their new Jaguar, or skiing in Aspen in their second home. My husband's a professor at Northwestern and I teach fine art part-time, so we're not exactly poor; but I felt totally out of these women's league. Well, not out of it, exactly. What I really felt, listening to them yak about their money and their lifestyle, was *bored*.

Addy
college instructor

Addy soon left her Mommy and Me, after her husband's teaching assistant introduced her to her own group, in a slightly less affluent area. Most of the national chains allow you to sit in on one class for free, to scope it out. Do that before you sign up—and when you're there, don't watch the other kids, watch the other moms: do they interact well with their own children; when they talk among themselves, are they focused on children and parenting issues? Or are they looking to see who has the nicest clothes and who's shed more of her baby fat?

Probably all mothers appreciate and enjoy the emphasis that many playgroups like Gymboree and Mommy and Me place on physical development, and what it can do for their children's growing bodies and minds. But don't overdo it.

*G*ymboree started out well enough, when the kids were all like six months old. But a few months later, it suddenly turned into the Whose Kid Will Be the First to Crawl, Walk, and Talk contest. I hated that. And just as much, I hate confessing that even *I* got into it, to the point where I'd say under my breath, "Yessssss! Go, Lucy!" whenever they'd roll out those Gymboree balls. Then Lucy wanted to win the sticker all the time, and felt awful when she didn't. And she was just ten months old! I'd better calm down before she's old enough to join AYSO or I'll be dead of a heart attack before I'm thirty-five.

Nadine
homemaker

There's nothing wrong with a little healthy competition but it's just plain silly to foster it among babies and toddlers, because they all develop at different rates. Girls tend to talk and walk earlier than boys, but boys tend to crawl before girls. One baby will start speaking at eight months; another won't talk until he's eighteen months (and then you can't shut him up for love or money). Considering how competitive life is in this modern age, do you need to feel that way about your baby? Plenty of time for that in nursery school.

If you don't like the competition vibe in your playgroup, you have two choices: either you just ignore it, or, better, you move on. Before you do, however, see if there are any kindred spirits who might want to move into a new class with you, and propose it to them. Leaving your original group is hardly the violation of a sacred oath.

Don't let yourself get caught up in the competition game. Get what you, and your little one, need from the classes, and cultivate friendships with moms you meet elsewhere.

A Class Act

Once your child is walking and talking, you might consider enrolling in a parent/toddler class, for kids twelve months to three years old.

What you want to look for in a good parent/toddler class are exactly the same things you look for in a Mommy and Me or Gymboree class: parents of like mind, a clean facility run by trained professionals, a good program that covers body and mind, convenient times and locations, and makeup sessions at no extra charge.

What the Other Mothers Know

But there's something else you should look for in a parent/toddler class, which you might not be aware of, and it's a biggie.

> *My* two-year-old and I attended a weekly parent/toddler class. When I'd occasionally skip a session, I didn't call to borrow the "class notes," or show up, frantically asking, "What'd I miss?!" One time everyone was discussing where their kid would be going in September, referring to "bridge this," and "bridge that." I had no idea what they could be bridging. I thought all the kids would be attending another year of parent/toddler. Ah, but what self-respecting parent allows her children to languish in juice and Cheerios when they can move up to push cars and sandboxes? My son was only two, and already he was behind the social-developmental-educational eight ball, because I wasn't up on all the right things to do.
>
> *Kim*
> *television executive*

So, what is bridging? Many parent/toddler classes have a preschool affiliation, often via special programs that "bridge" the gap between home and school, giving toddlers an opportunity to socialize with older children, become familiar with what lies ahead in kindergarten, and to prepare them—and you—for it.

Kim just happened to be absent one day in March when the director of the affiliated preschool came in to distribute applications to their bridge program. Of course, none of the other parents bothered to fill her in on that when she returned the following week, which is hardly a shocker, considering that all their precious tykes were competing for a limited number of preschool spots. When it comes to getting into good nursery schools and kindergartens, even that wonderful Other Mother you met in Mommy and Me can turn into an *other* Other Mother and sabotage you in what she'll swear up and down was simply an "act of omission."

Uh-huh. Sure. And there are no plastic surgeons in Beverly Hills.

Before you enroll your child in a parent/toddler program, ask if it's affiliated with a preschool; after you've joined, always ask the leader if you missed anything important during an absence, and keep track of handouts as if they were cash money.

Academic vs. Developmental

Before you even think about applying to preschools, however, you need to know that there are two different kinds of preschools: academic and developmental. The academic variety introduces three-year-olds to reading, writing, and math; the kids use workbooks, receive homework assignments, and are expected to maintain a certain level of academic achievement. Consider these programs the first baby step toward prep school. Of course, if your two-year-old is already reading, just give him this book and he can figure out for himself where he wants to go.

Developmental programs, on the other hand, emphasize physical activities, art, and dramatic improvisation (we used to call that make believe), while tailoring those experiences to each child's own, special developmental level. They also work with the children to socialize, and separate from Mom and Dad.

Where do you go if you want your kid to get a painless head start on reading, without having to buy her drool-proof spiral-bound notebooks?

What the Other Mothers Know

Most public libraries offer special programs to get toddlers interested in books. And most four-year colleges and universities offer reading programs in their Early Education Program. Better yet, why not just read to your kid? That's probably the best way to make him curious about what those squiggly black lines on the paper mean. Here's a tip from Donna for teaching your child the alphabet and the rudiments of reading: tape a blank piece of paper on the wall by his bed, and each time he recognizes a word when you read aloud to him, write it on the paper. He'll soon learn to recognize the word, and before you know it, he'll be reading.

Apply Early . . .

If you think that applying to nursery school and prekindergarten programs begins when your child turns three, think again. Some Other Mothers advise that the moment you find out you're pregnant, forget about shopping for maternity clothes and start shopping for your area's best preschools.

Okay, that's an exaggeration. But not by much.

In this country, we do not yet have universal public pre- and nursery-school education and day care, which leaves private early education as the only option; thus, the competition for admission is understandably fierce. (That's okay. Consider it a great dry run for applying to college.) With the great majority of all mothers of children under six now working outside the home, even so-so schools have waiting lists longer than the customer-service line at Toys "R" Us on December 26.

What the Other Mothers Know

Start looking seriously when your child turns two. Private preschools usually start their academic year in September, just like big-kid schools; therefore, their deadline for application for the upcoming academic year is anywhere from January to April. Check with each school by no later than September of the *previous* year to find out their policy, their deadline, and what age your child needs to have turned by the following September to enroll.

Sometimes new moms get wired into one particular school because their Other Mother friends with older kids have, or had, their kids there. Other times, it's simply part of belonging to a particular social set. And everyone loves to take the new mom under her wing and become her first Other Mother.

*F*rom the moment Kelsey was born, I was all set with a list of good schools, because my friends' and neighbors' kids were already there. How did I know what to look for? I just followed them. I had one neighbor, who said, "This is where you're sending Kelsey. It's the best preschool in the city, it's three blocks away, case closed." I was the happy idiot, so I said, "Fine, okay." Well, luckily for us, it *was* the best school—but that was us. For somebody else, who knows?

Beth

dentist

A school that's right for your friends' kids may not be the best fit for yours; however, it's safe to say that if you know some older-kid moms who are the type to do their homework, you should listen to their advice and then weigh the information for yourself.

Don't feel obliged to chase after the handful of hot schools just because everybody else's kids are going there.

*M*y husband and I were desperate to get Aidan into one of the three name preschools in our area. There was another one, but a friend told us it was just not on the list. But when all the spots were filled at the other three schools, we figured we'd check out Crestview. It turned out it was perfectly fine. Okay, so maybe they didn't bring in pony rides, or fake snow at Christmastime, but it was safe, and warm, and friendly, and Aidan loved his two years there. No matter what you call it, grape juice is still grape juice, whether you serve it in a silver cup or a Dixie cup.

Linda

journalist

If a school's difficult to get into, or immensely popular, and you have friends or colleagues who already have children at that preschool, ask them to write a letter to the administration on your behalf; often, it can make a difference.

And don't worry about filling out the applications. One good thing about nursery and preschool is that the applications aren't complicated; there's only so much information they can ask for, because kids that little haven't had enough time to build a dossier (or a criminal record).

. . . But Don't Go Crazy

We thought we'd seen everything, until we viewed a two-part episode of ABC's *Nightline* news show that aired in 2006, about the difficulty of getting two- and three-year-olds into the "right" preschools in Manhattan.

The producers profiled a well-regarded preschool located in the downtown area, which admits kids on a first-come, first-served basis. No application process, no interview, no name-dropping, no bribery. One afternoon in March, the day before sign-up for the fall term, anxiety-wracked parents began lining up outside the school in eighteen-degree weather, with sleeping bags and tents, staying there all night until the school opened its doors the next morning! We're sorry, but not even U2 tickets are worth that. Okay, throw in a backstage pass and a photo with Bono, *maybe*.

*W*hen Jamie was young, my husband and I felt an enormous amount of pressure and anxiety about getting him into a good preschool. You know the litany: if you get into the right preschool, you get into the right elementary school, and if you get into the right elementary school, you get into the right prep or high school, and if you get a combined 2,400 on the SAT I, you'll get into the right college, and from there it's just a hop, skip, and a jump to world domination.

Well, Jamie never quite got onto the fast track; he was an average student who wound up working for a few years after high school, bouncing around a bit. But at age twenty-three, he started community college, was able to transfer into a four-year school, made straight As, and has just been accepted into graduate school. He's done just as well as any of those kids who got into the "right" schools; he just took a different route, that's all.

Nancy
restaurateur

Does a child's path to academia begin in infancy? We don't know. But we do know that there's a legion of companies out there who want you to believe it does, so that you'll spend all kinds of money on their Baby Giga-Googoo Genius DVDs, CDs, and books. Please remember this: even Albert Einstein was a kid once. Do you really think his mother was showing him star charts of galaxies far, far away and singing nursery rhymes about time travel and string theory? Now there's even a 24/7 cable network called BabyFirstTV. Any idea what babies are doing watching television at three a.m.?

One preschool director we spoke with commented that the single biggest problem she sees among her students is being overscheduled; many of them literally have no free playtime because their moms have signed them up for so many outside activities. A three-year-old should not need a Filofax or a Blackberry to keep track of her day, or she'll come down with burnout before she even knows how to spell it.

What the Other Mothers Know

Moms, throw away the antianxiety meds and take a deep, cleansing breath (you'll doubtless remember that from labor). Yes, we know that things are more competitive today than ever before. Experts with far greater knowledge than we possess probably know the whys and wherefores, but it doesn't really matter. What it all comes down to is two things: whether or not you place your child in a super-competitive environment; and if you do, how you help her navigate it without turning her into a soulless drone before she's had her first Happy Meal. The decision is yours.

Our personal advice? Let your child have a childhood. A three-year-old doesn't need to know numbers (apart from saying "I have to go number two"), or be able to read Kafka. Lots of schools, private and public, now have kindergarteners and first-graders doing one to two hours of homework every night, crankin' up the ol' competition machine earlier and earlier. We're not crazy about this trend, nor are many educators, not to mention millions of concerned parents who'd much rather be having fun with their kids after school instead of watching them pore over their ABCs; after all, isn't that what they're supposed to be learning *in* school?

Other Things to Look For

Once you've narrowed down your list of preschools to three or four, make appointments to see the school before you submit an official application.

Apart from the obvious—location, credentials, experience, philosophy—what else do you look for in a preschool?

What the Other Mothers Know

The very first thing to look for, and the most important factor of all, is how do the teachers and staff treat the kids?

We spent a day at a preschool that had come highly recommended by several women from our Mommy and Me class; I'll call it the Sunnydale School. My son David, who was just two years old, went down the slide on his stomach. The teacher said, "We don't do that here at the Sunnydale School." Okay. The kid started to cry, I handed him a bottle. "We don't do that here at the Sunnydale School." He did something else, I don't remember what, and she said, "We don't do that here at the Sunnydale School." Finally, David got so frustrated that he went over to the windowsill and started kicking it. "We don't do that here at the Sunnydale School." I said, "I understand, but what *do* you do here at the Sunnydale School?" When it took her ten seconds to work up an answer, we departed from the Sunnydale School.

Corinne
office manager

Another thing to look for is the physical condition of the school. But that doesn't necessarily mean pristine.

*A*fter visiting several preschools that were obsessively spotless, my husband and I went to a small local school. It was basically this big dirt backyard. They had some good music going, the teachers had their shoes off and were sitting around on the ground singing, and the kids were making that happy-scream sound that only a delighted two-year-old can make. One kid was in a diaper, another kid had a hat on. It looked funky and warm, and we realized that if a preschool is cleaner than a hospital, chances are the kids may not have much fun.

> *Renee*
> *forensic accountant*

Yet another way to judge a preschool is by looking at the parents of the children who are already attending.

*T*here was a preschool in my neighborhood that I was checking out, and I noticed that a lot of the parents were older. Now, I know this is a huge generalization, but a couple in their forties with their first child are usually so hyper and so obsessed with getting it right that they can drive kids, teachers, and other parents insane. On the other hand, a fortyish couple on their second, third, or fourth kid, has got the drill down. These folks are usually pretty cool, and so much more relaxed. So, I discreetly found out which camp these parents at my neighborhood school fell into. When

I found out they were mostly in the multiple-kid, cool camp, I enrolled Lindsay immediately. The other bonus about older, multi-kid parents is that they're probably sending their younger kids to the same school they sent their older kids to, so, the school must be good.

Catherine
professor

Okay, nap time, everybody.

Be Yourselves

How to prepare your child for a preschool interview?

In a word? Don't.

There are dozens of books that claim to help parents prepare their children for the nursery school or pre-K interviews, but do little folks who've barely learned how to Velcro the straps on their sneakers really need that kind of stress? The stress should be yours; you're the one who's going to shell out thousands of dollars for your toddler to eat Elmer's Glue and learn all ninety-two verses of "The Wheels on the Bus."

Our Lacey is a bright, easygoing three-year-old who's always gotten along well with other kids. We expected her to do fine at the interview, but we coached her a bit for several days beforehand. "Share with the other children," "Tell the teacher if you need to go potty," and "Be sure to put away all the toys." We dropped her at the interview, and an hour later they called us, saying she was having "issues." We raced back to the school, and found Lacey crying in the office. She'd gone a little overboard on what we'd said about putting away the toys: every time another kid started playing with a toy, Lacey grabbed it and put it back on the shelf. This was an alternative school, and they decided that Lacey was too authoritarian, and turned down our application.

Karen

interior designer

If any school you're applying to expects students to stack blocks like Frank Gehry, fold a napkin like Letitia Baldrige, or share like Mother Teresa, do you really want your child to go there anyway?

One thing you can do to help your child make a good impression is to arrange for a morning interview, if at all possible. That's when kids are at their freshest. But sometimes even that's not enough:

*W*hen Stephanie was two and a half, we applied to one of those schools for genius kids. We had no idea whether Stephie was a genius or not; we'd just heard great things about the school and wanted to give it a shot. So, the morning of the interview we put her in her favorite dress, and were ushered into the nursery-school director's office. Part of the interview—it was a test, really—consisted of identifying objects depicted on flash cards. I'll never, ever forget this as long as I live: one of the cards showed an umbrella. I said to myself, *For God's sake, what two-year-old in Los Angeles knows what an open umbrella looks like?! Kids in England maybe, but not in L.A.*

That's like asking a two-year-old in Ohio to identify a beach. Of course, Stephie had absolutely no idea what this woman was talking about.

Helen
actress

What the Other Mothers Know

There's absolutely nothing you can do to prepare a three-year-old for an interview. It's like trying to groom a puppy for Westminster when it still can't figure out what to do with all that newspaper on the floor. Kids are messy, missy. They fight over toys. They eat sand in the sandbox (if it wasn't designed to be eaten, why does it look like sugar?).

The best way to help get your child through a school admissions interview is to let her know, whether verbally or through your attitude, that all she's expected to do is be herself.

Don't forget that your parent interview at the school is just as important as your child's. Pay attention, don't interrupt, and be polite—pretty much what you tell your kid to do, except *you* won't have to ask permission to go potty.

But applications and interviews are only a part of getting your child into nursery school. (If it were easy, you wouldn't have needed to buy this book.)

*W*hen my first child was two years old, I just sent him to the plain old little neighborhood day-care center my sister's kids had gone to. Later, when we were filling out Adam's applications for preschool, one of my friends with a boy the same age asked me which open houses we'd gone to.

"Open houses?" I asked. "What for? I already picked up the applica-tions and sent them in." My friend looked at me like I was insane. "You didn't attend the open houses . . . ?!" She had a list of schools, she was going to open houses, she knew everything. I felt like a total idiot.

Laurel

attorney

You *must* go to any and all functions the schools hold for prospective students and their parents. If you don't, the administration will assume that you're not sufficiently involved, which (to them) implies that you lack that volunteer spirit all private schools seek in parents.

Incidentally, the Other Mothers also have a deliciously sneaky method for bypassing the cyclical drama and trauma of school applications. It's called "feeder school." Instead of applying to one separate preschool, then to another for pre-K, *then* applying to elementary school, and six years after that, to yet *another* for middle and high school, they apply only *once*: to schools that go from pre-K all the way up through twelfth grade. Assuming that the child adheres to the school's academic and behavioral standards, she's set for the next fourteen years; and just think how much money you'll save on postage.

If you apply to more than one school, tell only *one* of them that they are your favorite. The admissions directors all talk to each other and they do not like two-timers. And send two to three letters of reference, espe-cially if one is from a parent already at the school. (Just make sure the school likes that parent!)

That First Day

A child's first day of pre- or nursery school is a momentous occasion, second in significance only to birth. In many respects, that first day is a metaphoric birth: your baby is venturing out into the great big world, taking his or her first step away from home and away from you. Most schools allow parents to remain in the room for a while that first day. But when the teacher announces that it's time for all the mommies and daddies to leave, the room suddenly turns into the rooftop of the American Embassy at the fall of Saigon: the sobbing, the clutching, the desperate pleas. Sometimes the children get pretty upset, too.

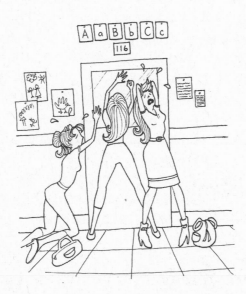

Many schools, however, allow parents to remain until the child feels comfortable with the situation. That's wonderful—if you're a mom who doesn't work outside the home, or you have a husband whose schedule allows him to stay. If you're a working mom, married or single, chances are your boss isn't going to be thrilled by you taking half-days for an entire week; and in some instances, you might lose pay. If you're rich, you can always send the nanny in your place. But if you're like most of us, that's not an option.

What the Other Mothers Know

If your child is freaking out that first week and you simply can't take the time off from work, then ask a grandparent, or an aunt or uncle, or a close family friend to fill in for you to make your child feel comfortable and secure. Each day, shorten the visit by at least a quarter-hour, until you've tapered down to just a few minutes on Friday. Of course, you can always make yourself so embarrassingly, humiliatingly, acutely, disgustingly silly that your child begs you to leave.

Another Other Mothers strategy is letting your child bring his favorite stuffed animal or blankie to school (in academic speak this is known as a transitional object). And each morning, when you get your child ready, allow him to choose the snacks he wants to bring, and to select the clothes he wants to wear (although you might have to explain to him that wearing a swimsuit to school in Montana in September might not be the best sartorial choice).

Some schools assign an adult buddy (usually, a teaching assistant) to walk with them; still others will encourage parents to drop their child off early to spend some "alone time" with the teacher.

But our favorite tip for a successful separation is the Mommy-gram; this is a piece of paper that you slip into your child's pocket or lunch box. Later, when she finds it at school and opens it, she'll be comforted by your message and know that you miss her just as much as she misses you. Of course, most three-year-olds don't know how to read, so it's best to do a rebus (a word-picture puzzle): draw a picture of an eye, followed by a heart, followed by the letter "U," and then the child's name (at three, most kids can recognize the spelling of their name). If you have a flair for sketching, you can end it with another heart, followed by a mummy. Put 'em all together and you get: "I love you, [name]—love, Mommy." It works every time!

Mean Girls and Bully Boys

Most of what kids learn in preschool and nursery school is how to deal with other kids; after all, they're not supposed to be tackling calculus or Latin American geography. Getting along with others is a skill we must all learn if we are to make our way through the world, unless we're a Balkan dictator.

I was in my thirties when I had my little girl, and when she started pre-school, I freaked out. Every time I'd see her start to fall, I'd go catch her. Or if there was a tiff with another kid, I'd run over and take her away. One day, the teacher came up to me and said, "Judy, I know you want to be a good mother, and Alex is a wonderful child, but she's going to grow up without any character at all. You have to let her fall, let her work it out with the other kids. You can't be there for the rest of her life." So I backed off, but it killed me! I'd have to close my eyes, because I couldn't watch her fall and get banged up, or get into a fight, but that teacher was absolutely right.

Judy
homemaker

What the Other Mothers Know

It's terribly hard to watch your precious child discover the hard way that not everyone in this world is nice, or good, or honest. But face it, it's good practice for real life in the real world. And in show business, too. We all must learn to negotiate with others, whether we like it or not. Sometimes that means dealing with jerks, so your kid might as well start dealing with them when the jerks are only one-foot-seven.

That does not, however, mean that there won't be times when you might have to step in.

A little boy came in during the middle of the term, and when I saw his mom, I did a double take: she was a celebrity. I won't tell you her name, but her son was a total bully, and bigger than everyone else; the other kids were afraid to play with him or even be near him. On his second day, he told my daughter, "If you don't play with me I'm gonna beat you up." Jenna was so scared she didn't want to go to school. So, I informed the teacher, and she said, "Well, this is so-and-so's son, so just let us handle it." Sure, they handled it all right: the next day, he smacked Jenna on the head and knocked her down! I was furious, and told the school director they'd better do something about it, fast. The next day, the boy showed up with his nanny. Meanwhile, the director was all worried that my husband and I were going to sue, or leak the story to the press. It wasn't the kid's fault; it was how he was being raised. I was impressed when the celebrity mom called us to personally apologize, but it was too little too late. We took Jenna out and enrolled her in another preschool.

Mary Anne
business consultant

It's a hard fact to learn, especially because it goes so completely against the grain of the democratic way of life to which we aspire in this country, but there are certain times and situations where status and money talk. However, remember that the bigger they are, the more worried they are about bad publicity. The rich bully in your kid's class may not be worried about showing up in *People* magazine, but chances are the school administration doesn't want bad word-of-mouth getting around your neighborhood, country club, or business.

My Kid Did . . . That?

Sometimes, even the most angelic child can stand accused of misbehaving. In these instances—and when it's your little angel—you need to ascertain the truth before taking action.

*O*ne night, when Hannah was in preschool, we got a call from a family, telling us their daughter refused to go to school anymore because of

Hannah. We were floored. "Did Hannah hit her? Did she bite her?" "No," they said, "but Hannah traumatized her." I thought, *That's a little weird,* but at any rate we went to see the teacher the next morning and asked what Hannah was doing to the little girl. You want to know what Hannah had done? She said to this little girl, "I know a joke. Hold out your hand." Hannah then said, "Here's your backyard. This is your house, there's your garage, now where do you want to put the pool?" The girl pointed somewhere on her palm, and Hannah dribbled a little bit of spit on it. Little kids who hear that joke go "Ewwww," and crack up. This was traumatic? We told Hannah to just stay away from Little Miss Nervous Nellie and play with the other kids.

Wendy
television director

There will always be parents who treat their children like they were Wedgwood china, ever-fearful that they will crack, or get chipped, or break. Usually, however, kids come supplied with their own emotional glue to fix that when it happens. But when you run across parents like these—and oh, you will, you will—play it cool and talk to the teacher. If these parents are as wacko as all that, chances are the teacher knows it better than anyone, so you're likely to get a sympathetic ear.

There Are Lots of Other Schools Out There—Really

What happens when your child begins a nursery-school program and things don't go quite as anticipated? First of all, do not panic.

*N*ikka was expelled from her first preschool, one that had come very highly recommended. We hadn't applied to preschools early, because we didn't know we were supposed to, so she started a few months into the school year. She wasn't allowed to separate gracefully, and a week after starting, the teacher asked to speak to me: Nikka didn't have . . . manners. Manners! They suggested we find a more permissive school. Nikka was two and had never had behavior problems. When I told my friend Diane what happened, she said, "Well, everyone knows they're a bunch of Nazis. Why did you send her there?" (There were obviously two sets of Other Mothers there: the supporters and the detractors.)

We then discovered the preschool at our local community center, which was way cheaper and wonderful—until Nikka's favorite teacher left and the entire place fell into chaos. Nikka kept saying she didn't want to be there without Bonnie, but we told her she just had to adjust. One day I dropped her off, and she came screaming into the parking lot, "Don't leave me here!!" I scooped her up and took her home. She's twenty-three now and still remembers how lousy it was after Bonnie left. Finally, a spot opened up at a lovely school where we had been wait-listed. It took a gifted and gentle teacher to make Nikka believe that school was a good place, not a scary, mean place. But he did, and she settled into a great preschool experience.

Ilene

What the Other Mothers Know

The first preschool may not be the right preschool for your kid, and it makes no difference who says it's the best school in the neighborhood.

It needs to be the best for *your* kid; that's all that counts. Listen to your child.

The "Experts" Speak

Sometimes teachers can be a little interfering. Or untrained. And please, beware of preschool employees who've seen too many episodes of *House*.

I enrolled my son in a pricey preschool when he was not quite two and a half. He wasn't talking yet, but we went to a pediatrician who's considered the very best in the Denver area, and he'd assured me that nothing was wrong with Carlyn; he'd talk when he was good and ready.

One day at preschool, two teachers called me over and said, "We think he's autistic." I started crying hysterically, then I jumped into my car and drove to the pediatrician. He's originally from New York, and he yelled, "What're they, crazy? You don't think I'd tell you this? Pull him the f*** outta there!"

Within the week, Carlyn was enrolled in another preschool, but I was still so angry that I went to see the previous school's director. I asked what these teachers' qualifications were, why they felt they could diagnose a thing like that. And she stuck up for them, which made me even madder. Next month, when we received a statement from that school asking for our next tuition payment, I wrote two words across it in big red Magic Marker and sent it back!

Barbara
musician

What the Other Mothers Know

Carlyn's teachers undoubtedly thought they were being helpful in telling Barbara their "suspicions," but let's face it: only a specialist in the field is qualified to make such a determination.

When a good, experienced teacher sees signs of a potential problem and expresses concern to the school's director, she may or may not suggest that the parents have the child tested. But sometimes, even then . . .

> *O*ne day, when my son was three, the head of the preschool called us in to say that he "doesn't have a conscience." (!) When we asked what he'd done to merit this observation, she said that he clearly seemed untroubled by taking toys away from the other children. Gee, imagine: kids grabbing toys from other kids! Luckily we have a friend who's a child psychologist, who told us how ridiculous that was and that human beings don't *develop* a conscience until they're six or seven.
>
> *Firouza*
> *environmentalist*

Here's the deal: if anyone suggests your child has a developmental or psychological problem, consult your pediatrician.

And don't drive while you're hysterical.

It's a Date

Playdates become a big part of a preschooler's life, because by that time your rug rat is sufficiently socialized to want friendships with other rug rats. But little kids' friendships are like adults' friendships: they have their ups and downs.

Sometimes, fewer ups than downs.

We've had some kids over that we never invited back. Once when Hedy was five or six, we had a little girl over. She brought her puppy with her, because she couldn't leave the dog at home alone. The kids were outside, coloring on the patio with chalk, and Hedy accidentally stepped on the other girl's drawing. The girl got really angry and told Hedy that if she did that again, she was going to tell me that Hedy put her puppy in the pool. I was just inside the house, folding clothes, and heard every word. I was horrified! To her credit, Hedy marched right into the house to tell me what had been said and that she'd done no such thing. I told her that I heard the whole conversation and not to worry, then told her she did the right thing by coming to tell me.

Trisha
homemaker

Unlike adult friendships, however, your little one's friendships aren't only with her peers but with her peers' parents. They come as part of a package. Sometimes, though, the complete package might not be one that you want.

Sean became friendly with a little boy I'll call "Matt," in nursery school. Matt was a sweet kid, but his mother . . . well, let's just call her intense. She was one of those nervous, obsessive mothers who won't allow her kid to go on playdates by himself; she *always* had to be there. I run my business from an office in my house; and my housekeeper, whom we've had since Sean was three months old and trust implicitly, supervises his playdates if I'm working. Well, when this woman insisted on accompanying her kid to every playdate, she expected me to take time off from work and socialize with her. And to top it off, she'd bring her one-year-old, who'd sit in her lap like a monkey, leaving dirty diapers and crumbs behind. To this day, this woman still accompanies her son to parties, and *he's now twelve years old*. When you invite Matt to a party—any party—you have to expect the whole family of four.

Suzanne
clothing designer

What the Other Mothers Know

It makes perfect sense to accompany your child to his first playdate with another kid, and well you should. But after you've met the other mom and seen that she's not running a meth lab in the kitchen, is it really necessary to stay with your kid every single time your kids get together? No, it's not. And if you insist on doing so, you might soon discover that little Matt's playdates are growing fewer and farther between.

But what do you do when you *do* like the other kid's parents, but you or your child can't stand the kid? For most parents, when you insult their child, you insult them. You may have to be devious in order to disengage gracefully.

*W*hen Rafael was four years old, a little boy in his pre-K class decided Rafa was his new best friend. Birthday parties with the whole class were fine, but Rafa did not enjoy one-on-one playdates with the boy. I didn't want to put him through an unpleasant experience not of his own making, but on the other hand, I didn't want to hurt the other boy's feelings, or make enemies of his parents. So I found out that the boy didn't like going on rides; even merry-go-rounds freaked him out. Rafa, on the other hand, can't get enough of them. So, any time the parents called about a playdate, I was ready with: "Oh, we're headed for the amusement park, would Charlie like to come along?" Pretty soon Charlie'd found a friend with interests closer to his own, and Rafa got a couple extra Saturdays at the park. I got sick of listening to that lame, tinny carousel music, but nobody's feelings got hurt, and that's what counted.

Jeannine
optician

An experienced mother understands that sometimes kids, like adults, just don't have that much in common; it's not a like or a dislike, it's simply a lack of shared interests. Yours is a loud girlie-girl who likes to organize My Little Pony races in the backyard at the top of her lungs, while the other child is an introvert who loves nothing better than to sit quietly with a book. Even when you make an effort to spare everyone's feelings, sometimes somebody gets an emotional "owie." Don't feel guilty about it; it's simply the little-kid version of "He's just not that into you."

Another issue can arise when you have close friends whose children remind you of *Children of the Corn.*

*W*e have good friends we've known since college. Unfortunately, their kids are hellions. My six-year-old, Jada, doesn't want to play with their daughter, because whenever she comes over, she pulls everything out and leaves Jada's room a total mess. Jada has several beautiful toy castles with teeny-tiny figures, and whenever this little girl came over, pieces always got lost.

My solution? We installed a high shelf for the castles. When Jada wants to play with them, we get them down for her, but when the other girl is over, they stay safely out of reach. Now that this same family's son is big enough to walk through the house destroying things, we don't invite them over much, and when we do, I try my best to keep everyone outside.

Barbara
realtor

Here are some more Other Mothers' rules of playdate etiquette:

- Arrive for the date on time
- If the playdate's at your house, get the other parent's cell phone number
- If the playdate's at the other kid's house, stay within cell-phone reach in case yours suddenly develops a bad case of the "come-and-get-mes"
- Don't send your child to someone's house hungry
- Reciprocate, reciprocate, reciprocate
- And most important . . . be on time to pick up your child!

Don't Play the Game

Do preschools foster competitiveness among the students? Well, that always depends upon the preschool. Some administrators and teachers will move Heaven and Earth to avoid it; others encourage it, whether consciously or not. What we've observed is, unless you send your child to the Kofi Annan School of Mutual Respect, there's no way to avoid it—because the most competitive people at any school are *always* the parents.

> When Ben was three and a half, he started learning his letters, entirely on his own. Suddenly all the other moms at nursery school were after me, hackles raised, demanding to know if I was teaching him at home—as if there were something bad and devious going on! They were resentful and envious a kid in the class was on his way to reading, and theirs wasn't. Pretty soon they were sticking their noses in my business, asking when Ben had started learning his alphabet, when he was going to play T-ball, blah-blah-blah.
>
> *Mona*
> *graphic artist*

What the Other Mothers Know

After wondering how she could defuse the situation, Mona decided to redirect her rivals' competitive energy: she volunteered to chair a school fund-raiser, then immediately asked the other moms for their help and expertise. Before long, they were all channeling their competitive impulses into raising more money than the last year's crummy, lazy, loser committee. Mona made some new friends, Ben was out of the spotlight, and the school got a new redwood playground set.

As of this writing, Stanford is the country's costliest private university, charging more than $50,000 for one year's room, board, and tuition. With prices like that, any parent who isn't a millionaire—and maybe even if she is one—prays that her child will receive a scholarship when the time comes. So, moms will tend to be competitive. Don't take it personally; just keep remembering there's nothing wrong with state schools.

MORE OTHER MOTHERS' TIPS

- If you start your own playgroup, take this suggestion from a friend who taught preschool for decades: Duplo Legos are the perfect toy.
- Make sure that any parent/child class you attend is in a clean facility, with well-cared-for, up-to-date equipment, and certificated or credentialed staff.
- Investigate whether your local public school offers SRLDP preschool (school-readiness language development program); parenting classes are a component of the program.
- If the private preschool you want is too pricey for your budget, do not hesitate to inquire about financial aid; virtually all private schools offer it.
- Check what stage of "potty-trainedness" a child must have attained in order to be enrolled in a particular school.

- When looking for preschools, see if there's flexibility in assigning morning or afternoon sessions to suit your child's body clock. Your lark might fall asleep in a class full of night-owls.
- Don't try to potty-train your child and "separate" at the same time.
- Don't send your child to school in an outfit that's expensive or precious; measure a good day buy how dirty she is when she comes home.
- If you need it, go home and grab another hour's sleep after school drop-off; it'll make you fresher for the rest of your busy day.
- If you prefer meeting on neutral ground for a first playdate, do so at the local park. It's a great way to avoid the awkwardness of not knowing whether you should stay for the duration of the playdate or just drop the kid off.
- Before a playdate at your house, ask your child if there's any extra special toy or object she doesn't want her friend to play with, then stash it away before the friend arrives.

IT'S IN THE BAG

- Baby wipes
- Band-Aids
- Change of underwear
- Change of clothing
- Change of socks
- Sippy cup
- Ziplocs
- Books (one for you, one for your child)
- A toy
- Pretzels
- Simple coloring book pages
- Sunscreen
- Cell phone with school's number on speed dial
- Wallet
- Kiddie CDs and DVDs
- Out-of-state emergency contact number
- Hairbrush, lipstick, and mascara, so you can look good when you suck up to the nursery school director

6

"Since You Left Me, Baby"

(. . . and Started School,
I Still Have No Free Time)

School is incredibly important to children's development: for learning, socialization, and keeping them out of the house for seven hours every day. We all want our children to succeed in school. We also want them to be popular, well behaved, and well liked. Following the Other Mothers' advice in this chapter may help you put your kids a few steps closer toward achieving those goals.

And if they fall a little short of the mark, well . . . just remember, when Bill Gates and Hillary Clinton were in kindergarten, nobody liked them either.

The Principals of Education

What criteria do private elementary schools use to judge prospective students—and parents? We interviewed several private elementary school principals to find out just that.

What the Other Mothers Know

Here come the entry requirements for membership in the phonics 'n' fractions club. In order to demonstrate kindergarten readiness, a child should be able to:

- Separate successfully from his or her parents
- Accept adult authority
- Follow age-appropriate directions
- Exercise impulse control
- Participate in a group setting for a sustained period of time
- Respect other children's space and belongings

Did you get all that? Good, neither did we. But it doesn't hurt to know some of these buzz words for when you're chatting up the principal at the interview.

Many private schools offer what they call Transitional (or Developmental) Kindergarten, which can be especially good for kids with late birthdays (not to be confused with developmental preschool—yeah, we know, we know). If your child doesn't meet the criteria listed above but you really, *really* want him to attend that particular school, consider this an option, regardless of age. Some parents are concerned about being held back for a year of TK, but they should ask themselves this: What's the need to hurry? Does it really matter if he's six months older than the other kids when he finally does enter kindergarten? Sometimes the best thing you can give your child is the gift of time. And don't worry: just because they're half a year younger doesn't mean the other kids will call him Pops.

If the principal interviews your child and sees signs of behavioral problems, all is not lost. Many schools are happy to accept students on a conditional basis so long as they sense that the parents are willing to work with them to help the child correct his or her behavior. Whether your child has issues or not, all school directors want parents to be active partners in their children's education.

We know what the private elementary schools look for in students; but what do they want to see in Mom and Dad? In the school's eyes, they're not admitting only a student, they're admitting a *family*, which means that the parents' interview is every bit as important as the child's.

If the private school you're eyeing is a religious one, you have to be willing to accept a religious curriculum. An administrator at a Catholic school rolled her eyes and laughed when she told us how every year during application season at least one parent will waltz in asking, "Yeah, yeah, but do they have to take Latin?" And parents applying to a Jewish day school should probably figure that Hebrew's going to be in there somewhere too.

Another principal believes that private-school parents are far more demanding than public-school parents; because they're paying tuition they feel they're automatically owed a greater say in the school's curriculum and operation. Such parents, he says, "wear their sense of entitlement around their necks like a diamond choker." Translation: these parents do not endear themselves to the administration. It's perfectly normal to have expectations about curriculum and facilities, since that is what you're paying for; but you don't really want your first-grader to be known around the faculty room as Son of "That Mom," do you?

Hurry Up and Wait

You've applied to one of the best private elementary schools in your area. April finds you breathlessly checking the mailbox for that thick packet that denotes acceptance into the inner circle. "Ohpleaseohpleaseohplease, take my child," you pray.

Instead, the mailman delivers a one-page form letter explaining that there was a "greater number of qualified candidates than ever before in the school's history," and that your kid has been wait-listed.

There's not much to say about waiting lists except "You have to wait." Or you can always try what an acquaintance of Donna's did. After her child had applied, interviewed, and was placed on the waiting list of a very exclusive private elementary school, she sent the headmaster a homemade frittata. Her child didn't get in. Someone should've advised the poor woman that if you believe the way to a principal's heart is through his stomach, you might want to find out first if eating mushrooms sends him into anaphylactic shock.

What the Other Mothers Know

Not to be flip, but a school can't be exclusive unless it excludes somebody. Why didn't Mrs. Yadda-yadda Frittata's daughter get in? Maybe the other applicants were simply more qualified; maybe there were more legacies than usual that year (children or younger siblings of alumni). This is certainly not to say you should immediately dismiss your kid's chances for acceptance if he is wait-listed; just the opposite, in fact, and this is true from nursery school through high school. Very often a spot will open up when a legacy moves away or, if the stars are truly in alignment, gets expelled. But go ahead and ask the principal's office where your child is on the waiting list. The Other Mothers' rule of thumb: depending on the school, if it's anything higher than number three, well, you should be happy with your second choice.

If you get word of an opening at your first-choice school right before or even just after the school year has started, go to the principal of the second-choice school and be completely candid about what has happened. Many principals in such situations will do the right thing—it is, after all, what's best for the student that counts, not the school—and give you at least a partial tuition refund so that your child can attend her or his first-choice school.

If your child is wait-listed and you happen to know someone who is connected to the school, by all means, ask that person to speak to the admissions committee on your child's behalf. You can also have your child write a letter to the admissions director, reiterating her sincere desire to attend that school. Just make sure that the letter looks like it was written by a kid, and not the editor of *The New Yorker*.

Incidentally, another option parents of any religious background might look into is Catholic school. Yes, many Catholic high schools are happy to accept students of other faiths; and their tuition is typically anywhere from 25 to 50 percent less than what the secular and the Jewish schools charge. Most Christian schools require all students to attend chapel, however; so if that's an issue for you, don't consider such a program.

There's Smart, and Then There's Smart

It doesn't happen often, but when it does, you've got to trust your gut.

*M*y daughter Georgi had just turned five and was accepted into a private elementary school for gifted children. In early May, they called us in for the post-acceptance interview, which her father and I attended, with Georgi. Several minutes into it, the director commented that Georgi was "fidgety." Well, okay, so maybe the kid had to go to the bathroom, no big deal. But then the director told us Georgi would have to spend the summer learning her letters. It took me about five seconds to decide that my daughter was *not* giving up swimming and outdoor fun to learn her letters and how to sit still at age five!

Donna

Donna immediately enrolled Georgi in another school that had accepted her, and neither she nor Georgi has ever regretted the decision.

Sure, maybe spending a summer learning the ABCs is some kids' idea of heaven, but it isn't everyone's. Donna listened to her own common sense and, perhaps more importantly, had summoned up memories of her own childhood.

Spend an entire summer inside, chanting, "A is for apple"? Donna's answer was, "N is for no."

The Competition Monster Rears Its Ugly Head

It seems like the older our children get, the more we're tempted to critique their performance and compare it to that of others. Except it's not all competition, per se; much of it is just general worry that our kid isn't developing on "schedule" (as if there were one). Our children enter kindergarten, and immediately we start sweating: "What if all the other kids learn the alphabet faster? What if they learn addition and subtraction faster? What if she . . . falls behind?!"

This mother learned a valuable lesson when her son started kindergarten.

*T*he first week, the teacher told all the kids to ask their mom and dad to write down how old they were when they started walking. The kids brought their papers to class the next day, and the teacher posted them on the bulletin board. It was all different ages, from ten months, eleven months, a year and a half, and so on. The kids got to see that little Johnny started walking at eleven months, and little Janie started walking at thirteen months, but *they had all learned how to walk in their own time.*

Several weeks later, on parents' night, all the moms and dads saw the bulletin board too. The lesson, so to speak, was this: just as everybody learns to walk at a different age, everybody's going to learn to *read* at a different age. The teacher did it to set everyone a model, so that if one kid was reading and another wasn't, it was all right. It didn't mean, "Hey, I started walking at eleven months and you started walking at thirteen months, so I'll be at Harvard afore ye."

Darlene

acting coach

What the Other Mothers Know

Like every developmental step and milestone, different kids grow and learn at different rates. If ever you're concerned that your child isn't doing what you think he or she should be able to do at a particular age, consult your pediatrician. And if testing is suggested, your pediatrician's office will give you a referral.

Don't forget: just because a kid is able to do something sooner doesn't necessarily mean she's able to do it *better*. The tortoise and the hare—ring a bell?

Supplies and Demand

When kids start school, they must bring supplies. But it isn't the supplies that matter. No, it's all about the backpack—and it had better be cooo-el.

Kids generally don't have textbooks to tote until they reach third or fourth grade; then, suddenly, they have geography and history and earth-science tomes that weigh a ton and bend their poor backs like palm trees in a hurricane. About ten years ago, a true genius invented the wheelie bag, the rolling suitcase that you pull along by a long handle. Those were an enormously practical, back-saving way for kids to tote all those heavy books. There was just one problem: they didn't look cool. Now all the kids carry messenger bags. Their backs are breaking, but man, do they look cooo-el.

What the Other Mothers Know

Instead of blowing your hard-earned money on the $100 super-cool-this-week backpack and another $150 for an office visit to a pediatric orthopedist, buy a second set of textbooks for your child to keep at home. That way he or she won't have to lug those books back and forth every day. If a second set of brand-new books is not within your budget, contact the school secretary to see if the school sells used texts. Or contact the parent-teacher association and see if they sell used textbooks to raise money; most schools do.

Magnets Attract

Most public school districts have magnets, special programs open to students on a city- or county-wide basis that offer the opportunity to explore a specific interest, talent, skill, or gift, such as the performing arts, science and mathematics, computer technology, and so on. Some schools feature more than one magnet program, and they are all usually highly competitive. So how do you work the system to get your junior genius in?

What the Other Mothers Know

In many school districts, you accrue points every year simply for applying to the magnets, even if you don't get in. Over time, those points add up. And although you think that your second-grader might not want to apply to a magnet in middle or high school, things change.

I never thought about my son attending a magnet, because we have a great local school. But a neighbor suggested we apply anyway. Her daughter hadn't shown any aptitude for math in elementary school, but in eighth grade she suddenly became a mathlete. Although the magnet she was attending didn't have a math specialty, she was able to transfer into a school that did, because she was already in the system.

Just before Teddy started fourth grade, I got a call from a magnet school with an open spot. We decided to take it, and Teddy's been there for two years now and loves the school. I doubt he'll ever be a mathlete, but if there's some specialized program he's interested in later on, he can transfer into it easily. Always keep your child's educational options and opportunities open.

Mitzi
writer

The Other Mothers also know it makes dollars and sense to buy homes where the best public schools are located, even if they're more expensive.

Let's say you, your husband, your four-year-old daughter, and your eight-month-old son are looking for a three-bedroom, two-bath home in a nice suburb of a large Midwestern city. You learn that Andrew Jackson Elementary, located in the lovely Whispering Pines subdivision, is considered the best public elementary school in the area. A 1,900-square-foot, three-bedroom, two-bath house situated within the Andrew Jackson Elementary School area costs $629,000. However, a mile away, there's a 1,900-square-foot, three-bedroom, two-bath house for $515,000 in the only-slightly-less-lovely Murmuring Elm subdivision, where Grover Cleveland Elementary is located. The difference in price is $114,000—a very substantial amount of money.

You'd like to save $114,000, so you buy the less expensive home. But then you discover that Grover Cleveland Elementary doesn't offer the same facilities, programs, or smaller classroom size that Andrew Jackson Elementary does, so you enroll both your kids in a private school, where you'll pay at least $6,000 per child for nursery school, and $9,000 to $17,000 per year from K–6. And in New York or Los Angeles it's even more. That adds up to over $160,000, and that's not factoring in tuition hikes. Do the math.

One more word to the wise (all right, a few words): public-school principals appreciate parents' fund-raising efforts just as much as private-school administrators do. However, they'd rather be assigned to permanent lunchroom patrol than face a posse of bossy Power Moms and Dads. They won't be impressed one teensy bit by your big-deal job title or your over-priced car, so lose the 'tude when interacting with them. Private-school parents are given a voice in faculty and administration hirings and firings; it might not be an especially loud voice, but if the parents band together, and if enough of them are big donors, the school's board of trustees will listen.

Be a Mommy Wars Profiteer

At most schools, public or private, you will soon discover that a divide as wide as the Grand Canyon separates the Mothers Who Work (Woms) and the Mothers Who Stay at Home (Shoms). The Woms feel—and usually are—too overextended to take on much of the volunteer chores; and the Shoms are hypersensitive that the Woms sneer at them for not working.

What the Other Mothers Know

No matter what side of the auditorium you sit on, play it smart and stay neutral in the postfeminist Mommy Wars. But just watch out for the Power Moms.

How to spot a Power Mom? Easy. Tell your favorite adorably cute story about your child. If the mom under suspicion immediately has to top it with an even more adorable story about *her* child? . . . She's a Power Mom!

While not all Woms are Power Moms, some of them do have demanding careers (or want you to think they do), and believe that their children's schools should be run like a corporation, with themselves as chairmoms of the board.

Power Moms will cozy up to the administration and the faculty to get what they want for their kids, but they don't stop there. They'll also glom onto other parents who are wealthy or influential.

*W*hen Joel was in third grade, I got friendly with one of the Power Moms, an architect. After deciding it was time for a bigger house, I hired her to design it. For a very nice fee. And then my husband introduced *her* husband, a business manager, to his boss, who then became his client. Big commission. Anyway, we all hit it off immediately and quickly became very close.

Then my husband's company went bankrupt, and our "friends" dropped us like the proverbial hot potato. When we'd see them, they'd give us this big phony "Hi, how are you," then disappear. Worse, their son dropped Joel as a friend, which I'm sure was not the little boy's doing. Eventually my husband started another business, and it took off. A week after an article on his new company appeared in the *Wall Street Journal*, guess who received an invitation to Power Mom's fortieth birthday party? Please, I didn't even bother to RSVP.

Tracy
homemaker

The only agenda Power Moms have is their own. They're quick to take credit for someone else's work, and even quicker to foist the blame onto someone else when anything goes wrong. Power Moms don't *do* so much as they *delegate*. Watch out for these users. They are members of the *other* Other Mothers team, who'll stop at nothing to make their children successful, especially if they can boss and belittle others while doing so.

Avoid these women, unless you happen to be one yourself. And if you are, be advised that we're on to your game, lady.

And then there are the Super Moms, able to leap tall swing sets in a single bound. These fearless, dedicated, ferociously energetic mothers will serve as room parent, organize the silent auction, chair the used-uniforms sale, and write the PTA newsletter. Simultaneously. Unlike the Power

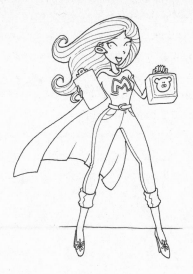

Moms, the Super Moms actually deliver what they promise. Nine times out of ten, you'll get very sound advice from a Super Mom. They can be annoying sometimes, these perfectionistas, but they get the job done. Ally yourself with them. Even if you don't do anything to help out, some of their shine might rub off on you.

But I Already Graduated from Elementary School!

In California, all elementary-school students must construct a Spanish Mission diorama. In other parts of the country, kids build dioramas of scenes from famous novels; scenes from the age of the dinosaurs; scenes from the life of the Incas/Maya/Aztecs/Dead Civilization of Your Choice.

But one thing doesn't vary, from state to state, city to city, school to school: it's the *parents' job* to build them. And every primary school in the country has its own urban legend about the kid whose architect mom or dad slipped a model-maker big bucks to build that pyramid/mission/fort/whatever.

The big question is, if all the teachers know it's the parents who are doing these dioramas, why do they even bother with the assignment any longer? We have no idea. It's one of those great unanswered mysteries, like what happened to the Lost Colony of Roanoke and where socks disappear to in the dryer.

Sometimes our inclination to compete can go beyond our kids' abilities and skills, and go directly to our own.

*W*hen Betsy was in first grade, the kids were given a Thanksgiving assignment: draw a picture of a turkey, then decorate it however they wanted to. They could paint, use food, feathers—anything. But the whole family had to do it; and the kids had to say which part Daddy did, which part Mommy did, etc. My husband and I agreed, privately, that this had to be some psychological test of the parents, but we said, "Okay, we've got glitter, we've got glue, we can do this."

The next week, I helped Betsy carry in our cute little cardboard-backed painting, complete with feathers from an old duster and dried beans for eyes. And then this other mother waltzed in with this papier-mâché turkey sculpture resting inside an antiqued box that was découp-aged with paintings of Pilgrims and Indians. And get this: there were battery-operated strands of yellow and orange mini-lights inside the box, to illuminate the damned turkey! Would you be shocked to learn that Mom's a professional film and TV set decorator with two Emmy nominations? I mean, give me a *break!*

> Cynthia
> health-care executive

What the Other Mothers Know

Savvy teachers can spot instantly which projects were executed by the 'rents and which by the rug rabbits. (Amazing, isn't it, how some six-year-olds can construct a perfect, to-scale replica of a crenellated medieval Lithuanian castle?)

Even while the teachers know that Mom or Dad helped—a lot—they still expect to see at least *some* evidence that the child actually contributed to the project. So, don't make their project too polished. Make sure there are one or two itty-bitty mistakes, like a tiny plastic machine gun in your *Salute to Prehistoric Man.* And for heaven's sake, don't throw away any project after it's been graded; you can use it for your *next* child's assignment.

Shopping with your child to buy all those little plastic trees, stegosauruses, pipe-cleaner marsh reeds, etc., helps get him excited about the assignment (especially if you throw in a visit to Baskin-Robbins for good behavior). If you go to a neighborhood hobby shop, you're bound to encounter an employee who's familiar with each school's projects and knows exactly what you need.

But please, do yourself and your child a favor: don't use such assignments as an opportunity to show off your own skills. Kids usually resent it when parents take over a project; they like being able to develop and show off their own talents and abilities. Even though they can't possibly do the job as well as you can, you have to let them try; it's the only way they'll learn.

A few more project tips you'll find useful:

- Hot-glue guns get . . . well, hot. Keep little (and big) fingers away from them, and use regular glue instead.
- Keep poster board, construction paper, glitter paint, stickers, and colored markers handy.
- Subscribe to *National Geographic.* Their science, history, and geography articles are digestible by non-nerds and they have lots of pictures, charts, and maps that can be clipped.
- Start saving shoeboxes. They make perfect dioramas that are small enough to be carried to school on the bus.
- Also save: fabric scraps, discarded dollhouse furniture, gift-wrap decorations (little plastic flowers, bells, etc.), pipe cleaners, pop-sicle sticks, chopsticks, extra buttons that come with new clothing, used greeting cards and old calendars, cellophane "grass" from Easter baskets, and corrugated cardboard.

Apples Don't Cut It

The majority of primary-school teachers are underpaid, overworked, and female (so what else is new). Private-school salaries tend to be even lower than those offered by the public-school system; and health insurance is not always provided. When a young teacher is out on her own and try-ing to decide between making a car payment or buying a warm winter coat, the last thing she needs in her Christmas stocking is a sterling silver, Swarovski-crystal-studded toenail clipper from Tiffany's.

What the Other Mothers Know

Many teachers have spouses who earn good livings, so it's perfectly fine to give them wildly impractical, even frivolous, gifts. Young, unmarried teachers, however, would rather receive something useful, such as gift certificates to Bed, Bath & Beyond, IKEA, Linens 'n Things, Target, Macy's, or Amazon.com. And if you learn that a teacher of *any* age is going through a divorce, assume that money is tight for her too, and present her with a practical gift or gift certificate.

*A*t my daughter's school, the room parents (all moms, of course) always get the teachers gift certificates from Nordstrom; they can use them to buy something inexpensive, then get the change back in cash, which they can spend on something they really need. A few years ago, Nordstrom stopped offering cash back on the gift certificates, *but* their discount outlet chain, Nordstrom's Rack, still does. It's a perfect way of showing your appreciation for a good teacher without saying, "We know we don't pay you anywhere near enough, so here, please take some money."

Geneva
sales representative

If there's no Nordstrom's Rack in your area (and we feel your pain if there isn't), present your teachers with a general-purpose gift card issued by VISA or MasterCard. These are very handy and every bit as good as cash; beware, however, that some of these cards charge up to $2.50 per month in fees until the card is all used up.

Better yet is the mall gift card, which you can purchase from the concierge at your mall; be even more thoughtful by purchasing it from whichever mall is closest to where the teacher lives. These cards can be used like cash at every store on the premises, allowing the teacher to pick and choose where and how she wants to spend the money.

Of course, it isn't required that you give teachers gifts; at some schools, it's even frowned upon. But if a teacher has done her job, or gone above and beyond the call of duty, you should show your gratitude in some material way. And if she's notorious for rarely giving anything higher than a B, we've always found that a brand-new fourteen-cubic-foot double-sided upright Viking freezer stocked with lobster tail, aged prime beef, and Grey Goose vodka is a lovely way to say, "Thank you."

The Hand That Rocks the Rolodex

The principal is the most powerful figure in school, right?

What the Other Mothers Know

Nope. There's one person even more powerful than the principal: the school secretary. *She* is the one who decides who gets to talk or meet with the principal, and whose messages make it into her in-box. Be polite to her. Flatter her. Ask her about her children, her husband, and her cat

Whiskers, whose photos she has plastered all over her desk. Let her know that you appreciate the many things she does. And when you're buying Christmas or end-of-the-year presents for your child's teachers, make sure the school secretary is on your list too.

Unfortunately, the school secretary—and the principal—is so used to dealing with whiny, desperate, or demanding mothers, that she can sometimes unfairly dismiss their concerns. If so, use your secret weapon. He's sleeping right next to you.

*T*he fathers have to be brought into the process, if for no other reason than they're male. Some of these school administrators, staff, and teachers, even though they're women themselves, are so sexist that when a mother comes in, they tune out and chalk it up to "just another overreacting mom." When a man walks into a school office? Whoa! There's a big flurry, the waters part! *He* gets listened to, and things get done.

Priscilla
human-resources director

Sad to say, but it's true.

It's like taking your car in for servicing: the mechanic believes all women are idiots when it comes to automotive matters, so he'll try to convince you that this doohickey is broken and that thingamabob is almost shot, figuring you'll agree to all manner of costly and unnecessary repairs. But if you have your husband bring the car in, and no matter if he hasn't the foggiest idea what a solenoid does or what a catalytic converter is, he's less likely to be taken advantage of. Does letting your husband take the car in set the feminist cause back a few decades? Of course; but it can also save you lots of that green stuff you work so hard for. You have to decide which is more important to you: making a statement to the school administration or getting your kid's problem resolved.

Ship of Fools, Carpool of Idiots

There's nothing better than being in a smoothly run, civilized carpool. A bad one, however, will put your stomach into a Prilosec-impervious spasm.

What constitutes bad, exactly? That would be little monsters who delight in picking on your child in the back seat. Parents who are never on time. Moms who continually rearrange the schedule at the last minute. Dads who listen to Howard Stern. Follow these tips to make your carpooling experience a safe and happy one.

What the Other Mothers Know

Scheduling: There are two trips per day—to school and from school—and five days in each week. Multiply two by five and you get ten trips per week. If you have a five-family or a two-family carpool, the math is easy. But when you have three or four families, it's a little trickier.

Three-family carpools: On any given week, two families will do three trips ($2 \times 3 = 6$), and one family will do four ($6 + 4 = 10$). Each week you alternate it, so that the family that drove four trips last week will drive three trips this week, and one of the families who drove three trips last week will drive four trips this week, and so on.

For a four-family carpool, use this formula: On any given week, two families will do three trips each, and two families will do two trips each ($2 \times 3 = 6, 2 \times 2 = 4, 6 + 4 = 10$). Whoever knows how to do tables in Word should be the one in charge of the weekly or monthly schedule, and e-mail it to the rest of the families.

The Monday grabbers: These are the sly moms and dads who realize that the majority of national holidays fall on Mondays; they "volunteer" for the Monday run so that when those days off occur, they don't have to drive. Adjust your carpool schedule accordingly, so that an eight-trip week is divided fairly among all participants. Or better yet, grab the Monday run for yourself.

Divorced families: If a kid is shuttling back and forth between Mom's house and Dad's in a shared-custody arrangement, put the onus on *them* to e-mail the other carpool families each Sunday, to remind everyone which parent will be driving that week, where the child will be picked up from, and where the child will be dropped off.

The after-school errand-runner: This is a parent who uses the afternoon pickup to run errands at establishments located near the school or on the way home. If this becomes a problem, tell little Ms. or Mr. Gottabuyit that your child now has an after-school schedule simply jam-packed with tutoring, music lessons, sports practice, whatever, and it's imperative that he arrive home in time. Make it up, if you have to. You're a mother. Lying comes with the territory.

Weaseling out of a nightmare carpool: If you can't stand it any longer but you don't want to alienate someone or hurt anyone's feelings, explain very sincerely to the other parents that you have decided to drive your child yourself, because those rides to and from school give you additional, precious quality-time together. Don't worry that you won't be able to carry off the act; just pretend you're talking to your husband.

And whenever you do drive the carpool, listen to the kids' conversations (without appearing to be listening). You'll pick up all sorts of information about what projects are due when, which teachers to avoid next year, and what mischief the bad kids in class are up to.

What if one of the bad kids is in your carpool? Remember, your car is an extension of your house—your rules apply there, too. So, if one of your passengers turns out to be a little pill, don't tolerate it. Start with a stern word to curtail her backtalk or, worse, her picking on the other kids. If that doesn't take, move on to a word with her parents. And if there's still no change in behavior, try the ultimate deterrent: have your child sit in the back, pick up the problem passenger last, and make her sit up front with *you*.

Uniforms

The majority of private and parochial schools, and many public schools and magnet programs as well, require students to wear uniforms. Kids hate it. Parents love it, because there's no wardrobe debate in the morning, which, if you have a daughter, requires a good half-hour struggle by the time they reach second grade and only gets worse as they get older. It also reduces the wardrobe competition that comes into play in middle school or even earlier, where the girls vie against one another to see who has the most stylish and expensive clothes.

Boys usually couldn't care less what they have to wear, unless you have a budding metrosexual on your hands. But if your little girl balks at regimentation, there are ways to compromise, which won't require professional mediation.

What the Other Mothers Know

Let your pint-size fashionista accessorize to whatever extent school policy allows; this way she can express her own style and sense of individuality. A scarf, a cute belt, a nice barrette, some layering—these can go a long way toward making a girl accept wearing a uniform.

But uniform issues are not limited to the girls.

We live in Washington, DC, where the school district can't require uniforms, only recommend them. Most younger kids like to wear uniforms, but once they get to be in fourth or fifth grade, they absolutely refuse to. Christopher is only in first grade, but I guess he's precocious, because he didn't want to wear that polo shirt and blue pants. Then, when I got him a pair of *Star Wars* underpants that he loved, I got an idea. I bought him eight pairs and made them part of his uniform. With Yoda on his little butt, he doesn't mind the blue pants.

Gwen
homemaker

Here in California, many of the private and parochial school uniforms are retailed through one particular company that has outlets up and down the state. A pair of pants averages $40; a white cotton piqué polo shirt, $30. Not exactly cheap, especially when you add it to those mega-bucks you're already shelling out for tuition.

Here's a sneaky ploy we know the devious among you will appreciate: if you have any flair for art, or if, like us, you're used to forging your husband's signature, you can create your own "official" shirt freehand. But if you lack artistic talent, do this: buy a $5 white polo shirt from Target or Wal-Mart, then Xerox a sheet of school stationery containing the logo or insignia they use on the shirts onto a thickish piece of paper or thin cardboard, making sure to enlarge or shrink the image/text to the right size (you'll have to go to Kinko's or Staples to Xerox, because most in-home printers can't accommodate thick paper or cardboard). Next, take an X-ACTO knife, or some type of sharp, small-bladed scissors, and cut inside the lines, like a stencil. Now place the sheet onto the shirt, use a Sharpie marking pen to fill in the stencil, and voilà!

Sharpies come in any color you could want; and they're permanent, so they won't bleed in the wash. Michele did this with her daughter's shirts, and not once in six years did any teachers, classmates, or administrators catch on.

Smells Like Volunteer Spirit

There are volunteer jobs at your child's school you want and there are volunteer jobs you *don't* want.

At most private and parochial schools, and at many public ones, moms vie like prizefighters for the title of room parent. It's a demanding job. You have to call and/or e-mail the other parents constantly, to remind them of upcoming activities, notify them of classroom policy changes, beg them to volunteer for fund-raising events, plead for donations to the parent association or scholarship fund, and scream for money for the teacher gifts. So who'd want to take on this task?

What the Other Mothers Know

While being a room parent is a lot of work, it has distinct advantages. The room parent gets much more face 'n' phone time with the teacher, which is an ideal opportunity to smooth any feathers your little darling might have ruffled when he likened her kisser to a baboon's butt. If you're a working mom, the advance notice of activities means you have time to rearrange your schedule to participate in field trips and class parties. And, room parents are regarded favorably by principals, which pays handsome dividends in sixth grade, when you ask for letters of recommendation for your little darling's application to middle school.

If you want to really get in good with the teacher but don't have time to be a room mom, there's one job you can do that teachers often get stuck with, so they *really* appreciate a parent who lends a hand:

Garbage schleppers get no glory, but they are highly appreciated in the karma department. And there's always garbage to schlep. After one particular event, the major planner mom assigned me and her (now ex) husband, a big-shot TV producer, to clean up the kindergarten room, which looked like Kansas after Dorothy's tornado. He sneered at the floor, then at the green garbage bags, and said, "Don't we have people for this?" Excuse me, but when you're a parent, you *are* "the people."

Ilene

Instead of volunteering to be an event organizer, show up on the day of an event to help. No politics, no commitment, just sweat and sore muscles after erecting seventeen easy-to-assemble tents for Monte Carlo Night. It takes less time than behind-the-scenes planning, and you're much more visible to teachers and administrators. Ha-ha. (A tip for all you early birds who cannot sleep after sunrise: if a school event starts early, sign up to be there at six thirty a.m. to help set up. You'll catch a big, fat, juicy worm all right: the principal's approval.)

If you can't be a room parent, be nice to the one who is. Many private schools actually mandate a minimum number of hours parents must "volunteer," so, if your schedule makes it difficult for you to help out much, or at all, a friendly room parent might cut you a break.

Get your child's father to do his share. If he balks, explain that where business networking is concerned, the schoolhouse has become the new clubhouse; many a deal has been struck between hair-netted dads over the steam table at the country fair hot-dog booth. If that won't motivate him to become involved in school activities, you can always threaten to withhold sex (assuming he's still interested in sex, and further assuming he's still interested in sex with *you*). And if he's an attorney, point out that if he, oh, just happens to stumble across a petting zoo for the Halloween carnival, with especially energetic little critters, why, one good head-butt from a baby goat could be worth its weight in gold.

You want to be active in the parents association but your work schedule doesn't allow you to attend daytime meetings? Then offer to work on projects that you can do at home at your own pace and discretion: doing the calligraphy for invitations, working the events, working as corresponding secretary, running the working-mom network, inputting the catalogue for the silent auction, calling parents, writing thank-you notes to donors— anything that can be done during your lunch hour at the office, or on weekends and in the evenings.

Whenever your budget permits, give to the parents association and the scholarship fund. Help your public school buy a new computer or Power Point. Ransack your children's closets for old clothing or school uniforms and books to sell at fund-raisers. Just don't do what this mom did:

One year, the parents association wanted to raise $25,000 to purchase more computers for the school library. I work long hours during the week but I make sure my weekends are free, so, when I was asked one day in January to help, I volunteered to phone the parents from my daughter's class with a personal request for donations. That Sunday, I sat down with my list of phone numbers and a short spiel I'd worked out to appeal to their generosity. I didn't want to call too early and risk waking anyone up, so, I began making my calls around noon. But no matter who answered the phone, mom or dad, I was curtly told to call back the next week, or got a hostile "Not now!" One dad even said, "Are you nuts?!" and hung up on me. This was the case with each of the twenty-three calls I made throughout that day. I thought, *Gee, has everyone gone broke all of a sudden and they can't afford to give, or I guess with tuition being what it is, parents resent being asked to give yet more.* Well, what did I learn from this experience, you ask? Never, *ever* call people for money on Super Bowl Sunday!

Gail
hospital administrator

This also applies during the collegiate basketball Final Four, the NBA play-offs, the All-Star game, the World Cup, the World Series, and any other major athletic event in which large men compete.

TV or Not TV, That Is the Question

A new battleground that often arises when kids start elementary school is the television. Many parents disapprove of their kids watching TV at night during the school year; they prefer they spend their time doing their homework, or reading, or playing, or, God forbid, talking with their parents.

Your three authoresses happen to earn their daily bread in this very medium, but even we support keeping the boob tube off on school nights or, at the very least, limiting the amount of time a child's allowed to watch it.

But how do you enforce the no-TV rule?

What the Other Mothers Know

First, bear in mind that there's a certain social currency that comes with the TV shows that are most popular with kids. Remember when *Friends* was on NBC Thursday nights? Come Friday morning, every office in the country would see employees gathered around the water cooler to laugh about what that wacky Phoebe did last night. Regardless of what you think about the value of popular culture, remember that the one thing all kids want more than anything else is to not be different from the other kids. What you might do is ask your child what shows he likes best that are on during the week, tape or TiVo several of them for him, then allow him to watch those programs on the weekend. Or use them as bargaining chips: an hour of TiVo for a good grade or a chore well done.

The TV isn't the only screen that our kids are obsessed with. There's also the computer, and video games. How in the heck can you monitor the time your child spends on each?

Here's what our friend Heidi devised, and she reports great success with both her nine-year-old son and her tweener daughter.

*I*n our house, we refer to it as "screen time." Each kid has a budget for any kind of screen time (TV, Game Boy, computer), totaling one hour on school days and two hours a day on weekends. They can split their time between one and another, as well: for example, they can spend a half-hour Monday on the computer, and a half-hour on TV. This way you know when they're doing it, what they're watching, and where they're going on the Net.

Heidi
homemaker

To paraphrase Gertrude Stein, a screen is a screen is a screen, whether it's on a Game Boy, a television, or a computer. And no matter what your kid's watching on it, the activity is, for the most part, passive. He'll argue like a Philadelphia lawyer that going on Instant Message is an altogether different thing from viewing a DVD, but you just tell the counselor for the defense that court is adjourned.

If you're concerned about what your child is doing online, there's a way to avoid arguments: let him have a computer in his room but *don't* hook it up to the Net. He can use his computer for as long as he needs to work on school assignments, play CD-ROM games that you provide, or play the games that came bundled with the computer. But when he needs to go online for legitimate research, allow him to do so only on your computer. Yes, you or your husband might be inconvenienced on occasion if the computer with Net access is located in your den and you wanted to watch TV or go online yourself, but it won't happen often, and it will give you far greater control over the situation. And probably prevent you from getting an unexpected C.O.D. package from reallycooloverpricedtoys.com.

The Other Mothers also caution against letting a child have a TV in his room. The temptation to turn it on after Mom and Dad have gone night-night is simply too great for the average kid to resist. Trust us, what he'll try to watch in the wee hours ain't gonna be C-Span.

Many schools, private and public, allow kids to conduct Internet research as early as kindergarten, under supervision. Teachers of our acquaintance report that most of their students start going on MySpace and using IM at home when they're in third or fourth grade. Just make sure that when yours do, they're supervised.

Number, Please

Just about everyone has a cell phone these days, but do kids really need them?

What the Other Mothers Know

Well, it all seems to depend on where you live, and your schedules. Here in Los Angeles, a.k.a. Shaky Town, most of the moms we know get their kids cell phones starting when they're in elementary school because they're worried about losing touch in the event of an earthquake. (Or a forest fire, flash flood, mudslide—we have it all.) Then we know moms residing in Kansas, Texas, and Nebraska—a.k.a. Tornado Alley—who provide their kids with a cell phone for the same reason. And if you're a working mom whose kid will be staying after school for sports, scouting, etc., it's comforting to know that if her lacrosse practice gets moved to another, distant field, you can track her like an electronic bloodhound.

Cell phones used to be strictly verboten in school, but in the last few years teachers and administrators have come to accept them as a necessary semi-evil. When we asked several elementary school principals for the lowdown, each of them said that while they are, technically, "not allowed," it may not be a problem as long as they're not using them in class or during school hours. One tip: keep your child's cell phone at the bottom of his backpack. It'll keep him from reaching for it to call Elliot to ask whether he thinks Wolverine could beat up Dr. Doom, and it's less likely that the teacher will spot it.

If you want to keep your child reachable but you don't want your little chatterbox making a thousand hours' worth of peak-time calls at ten bucks a minute, you should look into something like the Migo wireless phone, from Verizon. Features include a dedicated emergency key and a super-simplified keypad that even a little caller who doesn't know her times tables can understand. It operates on standard batteries, and costs only $50. Best of all, the phone has a maximum capacity of four numbers, which the parents get to program. Just watch out that they don't abuse the privilege: one day our friend Joyce received a call from her seven-year-old son complaining that his nine-year-old sister was bugging him. And where was he calling from? The next room.

Middle School . . . Already?

The years pass, as the years will, and now your child is in sixth grade. Ah, time has flown, hasn't it? (And taken with it your innocence, your natural hair color, and your money.) If you did not heed the advice we gave you in chapter 5, about applying in kindergarten to a feeder school, then now you have to apply to middle school.

This time around, pay attention, will ya?

What the Other Mothers Know

Most public-school magnets give admission priority to siblings of currently enrolled students. And virtually all private schools reserve spaces for legacies. It's a trade-off. A fact of life. Get over it.

When a somewhat-less-than-stellar legacy from a wealthy family is accepted, often his or her grateful parents will make a generous donation to the school. Those donations also go to fund scholarships. Scholarships for which *your* child can apply. Opportunities might not always abound, but they do exist.

And there are ways to hedge your odds on getting one:

*A*mong the middle schools and public magnet programs my daughter applied to was a private school that's generally acknowledged as the finest prep school in our city. We didn't think Randi was a shoo-in; she had an A average, but then so does everybody who applies to this school. And her standardized test scores, while high, weren't orbiting Saturn like some of the other kids' did. Still, we applied, and we made sure we included every extracurricular activity Randi had ever participated in, like playing the bass in her school band. Turns out the school was looking for ways to improve their music department, and the orchestra needed a bass player! Not only was she accepted, but she received a scholarship that covered 75 percent of her tuition.

Christine
financial advisor

Keep your child's options open and encourage him or her to apply to as many schools as possible, no matter how stiff the competition. Often, the difference between a yea or a nay hinges not upon a student's overall academic performance but on the breadth and depth of her other interests as well. Whether it's music, sports, or a talent for sculpting with dried mashed potatoes, put it in the app.

Whatever you do while your child goes through school, don't drive yourself nuts. You have children to do that for you. Do what you can, but remember this above all: your child needs you more than the PTA needs you. We have a friend who never served as a room parent, volunteered at her daughter's schools only when asked, avoided the Power and Super Moms like the plague, and not once did she suck up to the administration. The kid got into Amherst anyway.

These early school years are a happy, idyllic period when your child doesn't yet view you as a walking ATM. Sure, it's hard work, but it's also a great deal of fun. Make the experience as rewarding as you can by taking our advice. Believe us, we learned it all the hard way.

MORE OTHER MOTHERS' TIPS

- When you work with the PTA and encounter parents who complain but aren't involved, say, "I look forward to you bringing that up at our next meeting."
- To help your child learn about current events presented in a format appropriate for his tender age, subscribe to *Time* magazine's *Time for Kids*.
- If you allow your child to watch TV on school nights, make it contingent upon her doing her homework first (just be sure that she didn't rush through the job).
- Before your child goes to sleep, let her choose the clothing she wants to wear the next morning, then lay it out at the foot of her bed.
- Have your child arrange everything he needs in his backpack before he goes to bed; then, keep it by the front door, all set to go.
- If your child packs a lunch, prepare as much as you can the night before.
- Each day, when your child returns from school, ask if there are any special projects coming due. Put a calendar on the fridge, and note assignments and their due dates.

- Knowledge may be its own reward, but a tangible acknowledgment of a high grade never hurts. A privilege, money, or a special treat for an "A" is still a good carrot to put before the horse.
- Buy your child pens that have erasable ink.
- If your child is allowed to keep her textbooks, show her how to highlight important passages and information.
- *Never* argue with a teacher in front of your child.
- Mount a notepad holder on your dashboard (the kind with illumination is even better); it's very useful during the school year for keeping track of after-school activities, projects, and items for class parties.

IT'S IN THE BAG

- Baby wipes (face it, they're in there for life)
- Pens
- Pencils
- Post-its
- Kid-friendly CDs
- Breath mints
- Bottled water
- Tide to Go portable stain remover
- Wallet, with your child's school photos
- Cell phone, with school's number and room mother's home phone number on speed dial
- Hairbrush, cosmetics, and jewelry, for looking as hip and put-together as the Power Moms always do

7

"You Don't Have to Be a Star, Baby"

(But If They Offer You a $20,000,000 Contract, We'll Still Love You)

Starting the day your child enters kindergarten, every waking moment of your life will fall under one of two categories: she's either in school, or she's not.

From September until June, there's school (that would be your school category), and there's after school (not-school). Summer vacation? Not-school. Spring break? Not-school. Thanksgiving? Not-school—unless your child hasn't done her science project, which means it's really school, except with a big turkey and that yucky green-bean casserole.

Sports, music, art, dance, scouting . . . These are many but certainly not all of the activities your child will most likely get involved in, to a lesser or greater degree, as the years go by.

The very best thing you can do for your child is to view his involvement in these activities as a way to round out his intellectual, emotional, and physical development; to develop a team spirit and a *healthy* sense of competition; and to learn something that could become a lifelong hobby. (Not to mention, to get them out of the house so you can watch that Netflix movie that's been sitting on the hall table the last four months.) Yes, sometimes excellence in a particular area can lead to a career in that field, but that's not the point.

Your kid likely won't be the next Kate Winslet or A-Rod. Then again, somebody's kid has to win the International Tchaikovsky Competition or make it to the Olympics; who's to say it won't be yours?

This Sporting Life

Whether your child was born with a backhand like Serena Williams' or is a total klutz who can't even backhand his video-game controller, he should participate in extracurricular sports.

No matter which team sport your kid wants to play—baseball, soccer, volleyball, football—it will provide him with other skills that are important: it's a great socializing experience, it's a good thing to learn how to follow rules, and he might as well learn how to cooperate with others to achieve a common goal before their first spring-break road trip. Also, developing athletic skills can provide a child with self-esteem that he may not be getting at school.

But whatever level your kid plays at, with whatever degree of enthusiasm, always remember these three magic words: Tide with Bleach.

How young is too young to play organized sports? Kids can start playing with the American Youth Soccer Organization at age four. If your kid can run down a basketball court without having to take a potty break, can put on his shin guards right-side up, doesn't run to third base first, and can follow rules without calling the coach a "mean old doo-doo head," let him play. If not, keep him out until he's five or has better manners, whichever comes first.

But what sport should your child play? T-ball? Soccer? Basketball? The truth? Who knows. They're just happy to run around, and you'll be happy they're running around someplace where they can't break anything.

If you have a son, hand him a ball when he's two or three. Boys are born with "ball lust": if it's round, kickable, throwable, or catchable, they want it. More than the kid next to them does. "Gimme that back!" That's how sports were born.

As for girls, sometimes it takes a little more effort.

*G*illian is the ultimate arts-and-crafts, dress-up, "let's put on a show"–type girl, but my husband and I both wanted her to experience a team sport. When she was five, Jeff took her into the backyard with a kid-size bat and started throwing a rag ball for her to hit. Turns out she had a really sweet swing (his phrase, not mine) and she especially loved making up imaginary players she was sending home every time she hit the ball and ran around the bases. Next day she came running up to Jeff, holding the bat, and said, "Daddy, let's go rehearse more baseball!"

Okay, so she's never going to be a jockette in her heart, but she's playing Little League. And she *loves* that uniform.

Beverly

aesthetician

Heads up, single moms: your little boy is going to need a protective cup. Just tell it to him straight what it's protecting, and don't get cute about it, otherwise he might try to drink Gatorade out of it. If he complains about it being uncomfortable, you might turn on the ball game and explain that's why the big-leaguers are always adjusting themselves down there. You won't have to wait long to see one of them do it.

America's Favorite Pastime

Let's talk baseball. After all, it is our national sport. And it has the cutest guys.

So, what's the first step? Before you sign kids up for Little League, play catch with them! Or, better yet, get their dad to play catch with them. It's amazing how many parents are too busy to go in the backyard or neighborhood park and toss around a ball.

Baseball basics: you throw the ball, hit the ball, and catch it. But beyond that, there's another reason to play catch with your kid: safety.

*D*ean was on a T-ball team with a little boy whose parents were hyper-safety-conscious. They bought him a special batting helmet, which is fine. And he always wore a cup, of course. But they also made the boy wear this weird, Kevlar-type vest under his uniform—you know, on the one-in-a-billion chance the ball might smack him in the sternum. Unfortunately, nobody'd ever played catch with the poor kid, so every time somebody threw him a ball, he held up his glove, missed it, and it bounced off his plastic vest and right up into his face. Can you believe it? All that safety gear and they'd never bothered to teach him the *one* thing that would keep him safest: catching the dumb ball!

Deborah

events planner

In addition to improving hand-eye coordination, exercise, and enjoying the fresh air, there are other, deeper benefits, too, to playing with your kid:

Steve started playing catch with Shawn when he was two, and I think that's why he's a better player, because he got the catching and throwing early, and was able to build on them as he got older. Now that Shawn's ten, Steve spends even more time with him because of baseball. They're always together. If Steve's not taking Shawn to a batting lesson, he's assistant-coaching; if they're not watching the Seattle Mariners on TV, they're at a home game. Okay, it's probably an obsession, but at least it's a healthy one. Plus he's a lot less cranky. Shawn, too.

Maggie

textiles designer

All right, so now you're ready to sign your kid up. Unfortunately, this doesn't work the way it did for Charlie Brown and the Peanuts gang, with them choosing up teams on the sandlot.

Little League has a draft process, just like the big leagues. The coach dads get together, watch the kids try out, then do a round-robin selection of the players they want. Of course, that means the best players are selected first, and on down the line, until they get to that kid with the glasses who wore street shoes to tryouts. Now, this isn't as cold-blooded as it appears; it serves to keep everything balanced so that all the good players aren't clustered on one team. And, of course, each dad gets dibs on his own child, who's almost always one of the best players.

But you don't have to take on the responsibility of being a coach or assistant coach, or even learn the game, to keep tabs on your child's budding baseball career:

> *I*f you want your son or daughter to be a good baseball player, it's probably a good idea to marry a man who loves baseball. Or at least knows which end of the bat to hold. That way he'll become a coach, and your kid gets on all the best teams. My husband's from Holland; what do you do with that? Train your kid to become a speed skater? So that's how I ended up joining the Little League board. If you have a husband who's going to go out there and get involved on the coaching level, your kid's going to be treated well. But in my case, I found another way to play guardian angel to my son.
>
> *Kathleen*
> *marketing consultant*

Do remember, however, that there's a difference between being involved in your child's athletic career and being a jerk. One mom we know got so upset that the coach had placed her kid in right field instead of short stop she marched out onto the field and started swearing at the coaching staff—and the umpire, too, for good measure. When her tirade

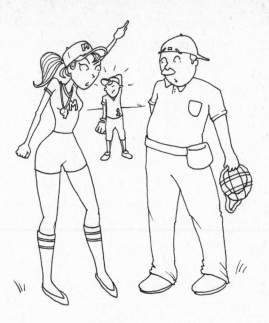

was over, her son was so embarrassed that he was glad he was stuck out in right field. There is such a thing as bleacher etiquette, girls; you wouldn't walk into a cocktail party and start burping the alphabet, would you? Pay your child the same respect; chances are he's more interested in watching the skateboarders in the parking lot than the game anyway.

The Other Mothers' rules of baseball etiquette:

- Never criticize another player, even if he just threw the ball eight feet over your child's head; his dad/mom/uncle/grandparent might be sitting right beside you.

- "Kill the umpire!" may be acceptable when you go to a big-league park but not when the umpire's either a retiree or a teenager doing the job for next to nothing. They don't care who wins and they're doing the best they can, so give them a break.
- Do *not* bring Fido to a game. When a kid's sliding to first, he doesn't want to slide into that calling card Fido just deposited.
- As boring as it can be to watch thirty-six pitches in a row without a strike, resist the temptation to whip out your *Vanity Fair* or laptop; you never know when your Ken Griffey Junior, Junior may be looking to the bleachers for a reassuring smile.
- If you have to use your cell phone, either keep your voice down or, better yet, take the call away from the bleachers.
- Don't litter.
- When you bring young children along to a game, please keep them quietly in their seats (and if you can really figure out how to do that, you can write your own book).

We've all heard the old stereotype about "throwing like a girl." Well, a lot of times, girls *do* throw like girls. There's actually a physiological reason for this, too complicated to get into, but here's the secret to curing girl-itis on the baseball field: *make sure that when your daughter throws overhand, her elbow is above her shoulder.* Then tell her to step toward the person she's throwing to and let 'er rip!

If you're not really into baseball, here are some key phrases to know so you won't sound like an idiot when you're cheering from the bleachers:

- The count: this refers to the number of "balls" (four = a "walk," which means the batter gets a free trip to first base), and the number of "strikes" (three = an "out") on the batter. The balls are said first, the strikes second. So, when you hear the ump say, "The count is one and two," that means the batter has one ball and two strikes. (Just think alphabetical order: "b" comes before "s.")
- Single: the batter hits the ball and advances to first base.
- Double: the batter hits the ball—a little farther, usually—and is able to run to second base.
- Triple: same deal but all the way to third base.
- Home run: duh.
- Error: when the batter's called "safe" because the fielders made a mistake. You're going to see a *lot* of errors in Little League.
- Double play: when the batter hits a ball with a runner on any of the bases, and both the batter and the base runner are called "out." (You don't want to know the details of how this actually works; besides, you will see very, very few of these in Little League.)
- The ground-rule double: this is a batted ball that *bounces* over the fence and out of the park, not to be mistaken for a home run, a hit that goes out of the park in the air. The batter may advance only to second base. So if your kid hits a ground-rule double, do *not* start screaming at him to run home.

Let's Play Some Football!

Most kids don't start playing football until middle school. (Jewish moms can just skip this section and go directly to soccer.) But they can start as early as age five in the Tiny Mites division of the Pop Warner Football Association league; there are also the Youth Football Association and American Youth Football. They even have coed leagues your little girl can play in. Because we all want our daughters to play football, don't we?

Football might look stupid to most of us, but there's a reason why Whitmore J. Foot invented the game back in 1868 . . . (Just kidding; actually it was invented by . . . oh, who cares.)

What the Other Mothers Know

There's a certain kind of boy who seems to have a biological need to smack into stuff (if you've got one, you'll know by the three-legged chairs in your dining room). Back in more pastoral times, these boys exercised their smack-into-stuff jones by chopping firewood and tipping cows. But now that most of us have gas fireplaces and bovine-free yards, these boys need another outlet (one that doesn't include invading another country). And thus . . . football.

Most Other Mothers suggest starting your boy in flag football, where the players wear cloth strips on their belts. Instead of tackling the kid carrying the ball, they just yank out the flag, and the runner is "down." There's plenty of blocking, running, and spitting on the ground, so the boys still get their chance to feel like Peyton Manning.

When Andy was little, he always wanted to play football. Begged and begged and begged. His first two years were flag football, but when he was nine and wanted to play tackle, I put my foot down. Too dangerous; no way. But after months of watching him wrestle with his friends in the house, knocking over coffee tables, and breaking his bed, I caved. Better to let him clobber another kid who thinks it's fun than to spend every weekend at IKEA. Well, he played football through junior high until he got it out of his system—and the kids got bigger than him.

I guess I should mention that he broke his leg when he was twelve. Playing baseball.

Nan
School secretary

Here are the basic key phrases you need to know in football so you don't yell the wrong thing at the wrong time:

- Downs: the basic concept of football is, you have four plays (called downs) to move the ball ten yards. If you do, you get a fresh set of four downs. So when you hear someone say "second and seven," or "third and two," for example, the first number means the down, and the second number means how many more yards they have to go to make the full ten yards. (In some kids' leagues, they simplify this rule so that the team has four downs to reach a particular line on the field.)
- Line of scrimmage: that's the imaginary line where the ball is spotted after each play. Neither team may cross that line until the

ball is hiked (thrown into play, although these days, they usually say "snapped") to start the next play.

- Offsides: when a player on either team crosses that imaginary line of scrimmage prematurely, he is said to be "offsides," and the team is penalized. (*Note*: offsides in football is *not* the same as offsides in soccer.)
- Personal foul: somebody did something really mean—even for football—like kicking or punching. If your kid commits one, skip the post-game trip to Baskin-Robbins.

I Get a Kick Out of You

We born-and-bred Yankee types who grew up on baseball, basketball, and football start teaching our little guys and girls about sports by throwing a ball to them. But people in other parts of the world teach their little ones to kick a ball; and when they move to America, their kids have a singular advantage when they join the American Youth Soccer Organization. So, as long as your kid's toddling, she might as well be kicking something that isn't you.

But since many Americans didn't grow up with the game, we might have to do a little homework for our kids' sake:

*B*ennett had never played soccer before, but when he was six, and all the other kids he knew were playing, he became eager to give it a try. The problem was, not only had I not grown up with the game, neither had my husband, Gavin. But at the first game we learned rule number one of youth soccer: the kids who aren't so good get stuck playing defense, down by their own goal—which is where the coach put Bennett. Meanwhile, the hotshots play offense, where they get to try and score goals. So, naturally, the coach and his assistants all wind up on that end of the sidelines, nearest their forwards (including their kids, of course) while the defensive players get ignored.

As Gavin and I were trying to play cheerleaders for Bennett, who was so far away from the action he literally couldn't see the ball, Bennett turned to us and said, "What am I supposed to be doing?" We said, "We have no idea." That day, Gavin and I signed up to become linesmen (they're like assistant referees) and learned the basics of the game. That way we could tell Bennett what he was supposed to be doing, and call the coach when he was ignoring the kids on defense.

Nell
homemaker

Most AYSO leagues offer a short course at night, which can teach parents how to be a line judge. It's pretty painless, and they're usually thrilled when somebody volunteers for this fairly thankless task. Mostly it involves waving a little flag and determining which team kicked the ball out of bounds. Plus, if you're a volunteer line judge, your child gets preferential treatment when it comes to playing in special tournaments.

Soccer, like baseball, is an especially good game for girls, because being big or tall isn't as great a factor as it is in basketball or volleyball. However, sometimes girls need a little help in one aspect of the sport:

*T*essa was a really good player, but one day she was chasing after a loose ball along with a girl from the other team, and as they raced after it, they smacked into each other—the way you see players collide a hundred times. Tessa immediately turned to the other girl and said, "Excuse me." I said to my husband, "Two words you'll never hear in a boys' game!"

Afterwards, we reminded Tessa that as long as you're playing by the rules, it's okay to slam into an opponent. Of course, I love having a polite daughter, but in sports, as in some other times in life, it's okay to be aggressive.

Patricia
musician

This will probably all change soon enough, once this next generation of girls have their own children; then you'll see a great many more moms involved in coaching.

Which reminds us: attention, all mothers with soccer-playing daughters. In AYSO, girls must remove their earrings before play can begin; in fact, the refs actually inspect their lobes to make sure the earrings are out. So, make sure your daughter doesn't get her ears pierced just before or during the season, because earrings aren't supposed to be removed for four to six weeks after piercing. (Sometimes, in school-sponsored games, girls are allowed to wear small earrings *if* they can cover both earring and lobe with a Band-Aid. Ask your daughter's coach.)

Here are important terms to know in soccer:

- Offsides: not to be confused with the term as it's used in American football. In soccer, it's when an offensive player (the team controlling the ball) is positioned beyond the next-to-last *defensive* player before the ball is passed to her. It isn't as complicated as it sounds. Basically, it means your kid can't just hang around by the other team's goal waiting for somebody to kick it to her.
- In touch: that's how they say "out of bounds" in soccer. (Must be an English thing.)
- Yellow card: when a kid's done something against the rules but not too terrible, like accidentally tripping an opponent.
- Red card: bad news. That's when your kid's done something really rotten, and it usually results in getting him kicked out of the game.

Finally, the goalie is the only player who's allowed to touch the ball with her hands. So, don't yell at the other side's goalie when she does it, or you'll embarrass your child.

Hoop Dreams

If your kiddie is a budding cager, the Fisher-Price Grow to Pro adjustable pole-mounted backboard is cheap ($40, plus a couple bags of sand to pour into the base), ideal for ages two and up, and will adjust from three, to four and a half, to six feet in height. Inexpensive enough to leave you with money to buy the kid basketball shoes. (You can also find kid-size basketballs at any sporting-goods store.)

If your eleven-year-old Shaq-in-training wants a regulation hoop, you can buy a perfectly adequate acrylic board to mount in your driveway, for about $100; or an adjustable-pole system for about $1,200; or a six-figure backyard court complete with smoked, tempered-glass backboard, eleven-gauge steel reinforcement, and, we should hope, a free basketball.

Key basketball terms include:

- The key: that's the marked-off lane beneath each basket, which vaguely resembles a keyhole.
- Air ball: a shot that doesn't get close enough to the basket to even hit the rim; also known as a "brick."
- Handles: if a kid has good handles, it means he can dribble the ball well.
- Hops: the ability to jump, as in, "Wow, that kid's got some hops."

Everyone Plays

That's the motto of the American Youth Soccer Organization. Add, "Especially the Team Mom's Kid."

Soccer isn't the exception, though. That's pretty much the case in all organized extramural sports.

*T*eam Mom is the usually thankless volunteer position that entails making calls when practice is canceled, organizing team parties, and collecting for and buying coach gifts. The one important perk is having the ear of the coach, to gently suggest, "If you want all those phone calls made, pal, my kid needs payback."

My daughter Amy is no Brandi Chastaine, but she's a solid player who's scored her share of goals. Yet when the All-Star team was announced, her name wasn't mentioned. But Harmony—who often talked back to the coach and went offsides—was on the list. What was the deal? Simple. Harmony's mom was Team Mom. Of course, by the time I graciously volunteered for the gig, Amy was into guitar. I don't think most garage bands really want a Team Mom.

Janelle
personal trainer

That's the upside to Team Momming. Perhaps the only downside is organizing the team parties at the end of the season.

*A*n experienced team mother knows the danger in offering options. The team party is an excellent example: ask when would be a good time to hold the team party and you'll receive at least thirteen different answers and one hundred thirty conflicts.

So, what I figured out was, you only clear the date with the people who really have to be there: the coach and assistant coaches. Less scheduling, less complaining.

Annette
administrative law judge

What if your work hours don't allow you to be the Team Mom, but you don't want your child to feel left out? Work the events (the concession stand, picture day, etc.) on game days; talk your boss or company into sponsoring a team; when it's your turn to be Snack Mom, bring the tastiest treats; and, above all, make sure you attend all the games. You might also join the AYSO or Little League association board; they usually hold their meetings in the evenings.

Snack Time

For kids, the most important part of every game isn't the scrimmage, it's the foodage.

When it's your turn to provide the half-time or postgame snacks, how do you know what to get? Well, start with this simple fact: your hand-dipped chocolate strawberries might draw raves at your dinner parties, but little kids hate homemade. They like crap from the store, in big, colorful wrappers.

So, how do you know which ones to buy? Ask your kid.

And how do you know which snacks to stay away from? Look at the field at the end of each Saturday and see what the kids threw away. We're betting it's the orange slices and anything with oatmeal in it.

Fruit roll-ups are a pretty good compromise. They're sort of candy, which makes the kids happy, and sort of fruit, which will get you fewer glares from the Psycho Tofu Moms.

If you really do want to be more health-conscious, here's a way to serve fruit that'll be a big hit with your little athlete and her teammates: buy two pounds of seedless grapes, both red and green. The night before the game, wash them, dry them *thoroughly*, and pluck them off the stems. Throw them into a baggie, and freeze them. Keep them frozen until the game starts; by half-time, they're like bite-size Popsicles.

When it's your turn to bring drinks for the kids, bear this in mind:

I once brought a cooler full of Capri-Sun fruit-juice drinks for half-time. You know, they come in a pouch with a little straw attached, which you poke down into the pouch. It probably took the first kid about ten seconds to figure out that when you squeeze the pouch, the juice squirts out the straw. Instant squirt-gun! Before the coach knew what was happening, his well-disciplined team had turned into fruit-flavored laser-tag fiends, who wound up really thirsty for the second half. So, now I buy drinks that come in plastic bottles with lids.

Tina

landscaper

Take comfort in knowing that whatever you bring when it's your turn to provide the snacks, you'll never make everybody happy. Basically, it's this: do you want to impress the kids, or do you want to impress the other moms? If it's your child's peers you're most concerned with, leave the carrot juice and the edamame beans at home. (And for everybody's peace of mind, leave the peanuts and peanut butter at home, too.)

They Can't All Be Pros

When your child participates in sports, be prepared to interact with plenty of parents who are so obsessed with their kids' athletic achievement they're like Lady Macbeth with a seat cushion. Whence this less-than-magnificent obsession?

What the Other Mothers Know

It's not pathological in origin but financial. These parents want their kids to win athletic scholarships, or what we call jockerships. College has become so absurdly expensive that parents want their kids' funding opportunities to be as broad as possible. And it's not just to college, either. Big-time sports has so corrupted athletics that its influence has seeped down to the secondary level as well, with kids competing for scholarships to the top prep schools.

What's the best way to handle dads who think they're coaching the BoSox instead of the smelly sox? They may call it Little League, but sometimes it's more like Big Ego.

If you feel strongly that your child's coach is not acting in the team's best interest, first talk to the coach about your concerns. If he's too gonzo to see reason, talk to the other parents. If they agree, and you speak to him on behalf of the group, that should get through to the Tommy La Sorda wannabe; he won't want to leave work early and lug equipment to a practice field where nobody showed up but he and his kid. If all else fails, contact the league commissioner. But the best way to get rid of bad coaches is to become one yourself (a good one, that is), or an assistant coach. As part of the organization, you can help prevent your kid's weekly game from turning into the Series, and give it back to the kids; sometimes they're more mature than their parents.

It's All How You Play the Game

As the Tom Hanks character said in *A League of Their Own,* there's no crying in baseball. Nor is there crying in soccer, basketball, volleyball, football, field hockey, ice hockey, lacrosse, skiing, swimming, weight lifting, ice skating, and probably curling. That is, unless somebody gets hurt.

If your child is injured during a game and is in physical pain, that's one thing; but if a kid's sniveling because she didn't make it to third, or Coach benched him the last quarter, nip it in the bud.

*T*he first year my husband, Tony, coached Little League, one of the boys obviously had never played sports before. When he'd catch the ball, he'd turn to his mom in the bleachers and whine that his hand hurt. When he ran to first base, he'd whine that his feet hurt. During one practice, Tony found him whining and fidgeting. Tony asked him what the matter was, and the kid started sniffling, "My hat hurts!" As Tony patiently adjusted the kid's hatband, I figured out the problem, and invited his mom to get some coffee with me. Tony told me later that the boy finished the rest of their drills without a single complaint. When his mom wasn't there to whine to, he "sucked it up," as the boys say.

Monica
actuary

One reason for playing a sport is to learn the difference between being uncomfortable and being hurt. If you play a sport and your muscles burn, that means you're getting stronger, not weaker. Kids—especially kids who sit in front of computers and televisions all day—need to learn how much more their bodies can do than they ever realized.

Sports are also important for learning how to handle life's little disappointments. Some famous college football coach once said something like this: "Everybody thinks winning builds character. Winning builds ego. *Losing* builds character."

No matter how terrific a player your kid is, he will have wins and losses in life. What better way to accept that than in this relatively benign environment?

C'mon, it's only a game.

> We don't wish to give individual sports short shrift here: ice skating, horseback riding, martial arts, golf, tennis, archery, skiing, and swimming are also worthwhile. They don't teach teamwork per se, but they do teach personal responsibility and instill an awareness of the importance and fun of physical activity. Even golf, believe it or not, is a great game for little kids (it sure didn't hurt Tiger Woods). And, best of all, you never have to be Team Mom.

If It's Tuesday, It Must Be Piano

Today's kids have after-school schedules stuffed tighter than Emeril's Cajun andouille sausages. The need to impress college admissions committees with stellar grades and Renaissance man–worthy extracurricular activities has obliged parents to seek private instruction to augment their kids' education.

Most mothers want to make sure that somewhere in the midst of that jam-packed agenda is musical education. After all, is a kid really educated if he can't appreciate both Green Day *and* Gershwin?

What the Other Mothers Know

Many parents love the convenience of having a piano-slash-guitar-slash-whatever teacher come to the house, and many teachers are happy to do so; just expect to pay about 15–20 percent more for the lesson.

However, if you discover you're raising the next Yo-Yo Ma, be aware that the most in-demand teachers may require that lessons be taken in their studio.

How do you find a good music instructor who's not too expensive? One of the eternal truths of the music business is that most musicians need money, so even the most talented will take on private students. Our friend Claudia, an advertising copywriter, found a fantastic piano teacher for her son when she was at the recording session for a commercial she'd written. You may not be in the music business yourself, but the next time you're at a wedding, bar mitzvah, or the piano lounge at the Holiday Inn and you hear a terrific band, pianist, or string quartet, put out the feelers; you never know.

Another fine resource for good music teachers is the faculty at your local high school. The only people who need money more than musicians are teachers, so there's a pretty good chance you'll find someone who not only knows music but knows how to work with kids. And don't forget the music store where you bought your child's instrument; they always have plenty of instructors to recommend.

But the big issue with kids and music lessons is, how to make them practice? If your child's a prodigy, it's not an issue; but when most kids figure out that playing a musical instrument requires actual work and study, they start finding other things to do. How do you make them stick with it?

*T*im enjoyed his piano lessons, so there was rarely any issue with getting him to practice. But one day, when he was twelve, he said, "Mom, I don't want to play piano anymore." My first instinct was to say, "Get your butt back on that bench and practice." Which I did, the first few times. Of course, it turned into a titanic battle of wills. Then I realized that either he thought piano wasn't cool anymore or he was just tired of it, or both, so I bought him a used electric guitar. He jumped at this. He thought he'd won the battle, but the important thing was, I'd kept him interested in music. And now, every other afternoon, I hear him at the piano, picking out a song for his band. If he can ever form one.

Lorna
homemaker

Another way to get music into kids' lives is by joining a chorus or glee club. Some schools offer them, and many churches and synagogues have children's choirs.

*W*e found a community chorus for Nikka, which she joined in the fifth grade (she could have started earlier if one of the Other Mothers had told us about it!). Being a member of the Los Angeles Children's Chorus was one of the most valuable experiences of her life. She toured internationally, sang at the Sydney Opera House, the Hollywood Bowl, on the *Tonight Show,* at the L.A. Opera . . . it was fantastic. A serious chorus like LACC is time-consuming and tuition-based (although scholarships are available), but Nikka not only learned about music, she also learned about teamwork, discipline, and the rewards of hard work. Everything but how to make her bed.

Ilene

Virtually every major city in the United States has a children's chorus; typically, students are eligible from grades three through twelve, and most choruses require an audition.

Art for Kid's Sake

Art, like music, should be a part of every child's life. Some day you're going to walk through a museum with them, and it's always a lot more pleasant experience for you if they're not bored.

What the Other Mothers Know

To really appreciate art, you need to have a working knowledge of how the artist got his or her vision up there on that canvas or pedestal. If you didn't know the rules of soccer, it would just look like a bunch of people in garish shorts and ugly shoes running around in the grass for no reason. Visit a gallery with a kid who knows nothing about art, and, whether it's representational or abstract, it's just pictures of fruit or squiggly lines to her. That's because she doesn't know the rules. So, how do you turn your uncultured Crayola chewer into Sister Wendy?

When your little ones are too little to do much more than make a mess, find a place where you don't have to worry about it. Put down a plastic drop cloth in one room of your house and buy a set of water-based paints and construction paper to let them express themselves. What they produce won't be hung anywhere but on your fridge, but your child will develop a basic sense of form, making shapes, using color, and mixing colors to make new ones. In every city, you'll find private art studios for kids, where they can basically do the same thing, only somebody else will clean up the mess. (Check out your local Y to start.)

When kids develop sufficient motor skills to control a pencil or piece of charcoal, they need to learn how to draw something recognizable before heading back into Abstract City. After a while, just making colored smears on a piece of paper gets boring.

When Dane was seven, I wanted to give him a background in art, even though he was more of a sports and video-games kind of kid. But I talked him into going to at least one lesson from a teacher I'd heard was terrific. In the first twenty minutes, she taught all twelve kids how to draw a sneaker, by breaking the object down into its simple component shapes. Dane was so thrilled and impressed with his own creation, he happily went back to the class every Wednesday afternoon. I don't know whether he'll become the next Julian Schnabel, but he's learned a lot. And he draws the coolest, scariest Halloween characters for all his friends.

Carole
quilter

If it's difficult to get your child into drawing or painting, try getting her interested in making three-dimensional art. Almost every kid loves to play with clay, but real modeling clay is oily, messy, and expensive; and

Play-Doh cracks when it dries. So, we recommend Sculpey, a pliable polymer clay that feels like the real deal but is a lot more kid-friendly. It comes in bright colors, you don't have to knead it to soften it, and it's easily baked in a toaster oven to kiln your child's finished product. You'll wind up with so many adorable refrigerator magnets, you'll have to start putting them on your washer, your dryer, your stove . . .

Colored pencils are better for budding artists than crayons or markers, because they can be erased. If a child starts to feel each line she draws is permanent, it can restrict her creativity.

Take a pad and colored pencils to the art museum and have your child do his own version of a Van Gogh or Picasso.

Find postcards or prints of famous paintings on exhibit at the museum, then, when you tour the exhibit, see if the kids can match the picture to the actual artwork.

When your child plays with one of those craft kits with tiny beads, sequins, or buttons, have her use it outside, or at least on a surface that can be *swept*, not vacuumed.

Buy the cheaper sketch pads that come in big tablets; as brilliant as we're sure your child's work is, she doesn't need canvas or heavy-bond paper to draw a stick figure of your dog sniffing a tree.

On Your Toes

It seems like every little girl has dreamed of being a ballet dancer. Even a few little boys. (If your son has a natural affinity for grand jetés, you might have the next Billy Elliot.)

Any dad who thinks ballet is just a cute little hobby for his darling daughter ought to try jumping three feet in the air and landing on the ball of his foot. When he gets out of surgery, he'll probably agree that ballet is hard work. Belly up to the barre, boys.

What the Other Mothers Know

The competition to become a professional ballerina is every bit as hard as that to become a professional athlete—probably harder, since there are fewer ballet companies in this country than there are professional sports franchises. You may be perfectly satisfied for your daughter to learn about the art of the dance and get great exercise, but not every mother you meet in dance class is.

*Ü*ber Dance Moms live for their child's dancing. They drive their daughters to and from lessons, wash and iron their dance clothes, sew their pointe shoes, and provide creative Tupperware meals. Some are savagely competitive; others are nice as can be. But either way, you have to wonder, *Do they have a life?*

My first instinct was, *I don't have time to be like these women.* But of course I wanted Jenny to keep up, so I befriended a couple of the Über Dance Moms. I soon found out everything about where to get the best leotards and where the summer dance programs are. For a working mom, these women can be a godsend; but just stay on their good side. And *always* be excited when their kid is a mouse in *The Nutcracker.* "My goodness, the way Miranda rubbed her paws during the pas de deux was so convincing!"

Frances
stockbroker

All the World's a Stage

Many a stage mother is born from the school play, talent show, or fall pageant. Stage mothers are a hybrid of Super Mom, Power Mom, and Mama Rose. Sometimes they're so arrogant they won't deign to let their kids appear in the production unless they get the lead, and other times they'll simply do anything to put their child in the spotlight.

*H*eather is a dancer and into the performing arts, and one semester she couldn't get involved in school productions because of her dance schedule. But that spring, when a particular school production came up, she decided to audition. When I asked the drama teacher about tryouts, she was surprised. "But I heard that Heather can't join us because of her dance schedule." I asked who'd told her that, and learned that the mother of the girl who'd been competing with Heather since kindergarten had taken it upon herself to "inform" the drama teacher that Heather was unavailable.

Lilly
marketing director

What the Other Mothers Know

The surest way *not* to help your child is to interfere with the teachers' casting process. They've seen firsthand how connections and influence can land untalented performers roles they don't deserve; consequently, they will not tolerate rule-bending or unfair advantages. (Incidentally, Lilly's daughter tried out, got the lead, and the other mother's daughter found herself painting scenery.)

*W*hen Abby was in fifth grade at our synagogue's day school, I volunteered to stage-manage the Old Testament pageant, which put me in charge of fifty eleven-year-old boys loathe to appear on stage in knee-length robes, and fifty eleven-year-old girls having bad-hair days of literally biblical proportions. Ten minutes before curtain on opening night, a Power Mom, who found the coat of many colors unflattering to her little Joseph, showed up backstage with historically accurate costumes for all the kids.

I pointed out that the school had already provided perfectly good costumes, but she blew me off and began handing out costumes, ordering the children to change into them.

Michele

An Other Mom saw what was happening; she quietly went out into the house, brought the principal backstage, and had *her* read Power Mom the riot act. The show went on, the kids were troupers, and little Joseph emoted just fine in polyester. Whenever a Power Mom tries to pull rank on you at a school-sponsored event, no matter what it is, just take yourself out of the equation and allow the proper authority figure to set her straight.

But when *you're* the authority figure and you've got to deal with the mother of all stage mothers, what do you do?

*B*en and I were in charge of the variety show at our daughter's day school for years. Producing these events comes under the heading of "No Good Deed Goes Unpunished." Once, a particularly obnoxious dad demanded that I give his daughter extra time for her seven-minute clarinet solo. I snapped. I handed him the clipboard, the stopwatch, and the list of acts, and told him to take over. Most Power Parents are used to dealing with frightened employees and intimidated sales clerks; they don't know how to handle an unpaid volunteer. What was he going to do, fire me? He agreed I was doing a fine job and slunk off the stage.

Ilene

The Other Mothers' Rules of Auditorium Etiquette:

- Don't be a seat hog and rope off a row of seats for friends and relatives who may not show for the performance.
- If you want to videotape your child's performance, be mindful of where you stand and don't block others' view of the stage. (To be even less obtrusive, use a smaller monopod for your camera rather than a tripod.)
- Turn off your cell phone.
- If you bring little children to the show, please be prepared to take them out of the auditorium if they start to fuss. Young performers

are nervous enough without having to worry about being upstaged by a three-year-old yelling, "I gotta go potty!"

Be Prepared!

Scouting, Girl or Boy, is an excellent way for kids to learn a healthy respect for that biggest Other Mother of all: Mother Nature.

Volunteer to be a Cubs or Boy Scouts den mother if you're the hardy, outdoor type. If you're not, volunteer your husband.

Most moms don't go on the overnight camping trips, but they certainly get stuck with the packing for them. And it's just a little bit different from packing a suitcase.

*F*or Quentin's first overnight backpacking trip, I was clueless. The scoutmaster had given me a long list of all the things he was supposed to take, but he didn't write down how you were supposed to pack it. I just naturally did it like a grocery bag: heavy things on the bottom, light things on the top.

When the kids came back Sunday morning, Quentin's pack was a mess and he had a kid's version of a grandpa walk. The scoutmaster explained they'd had to repack Quentin's pack in the middle of the hike. Turns out that the heavy gear should be at the *top* of the pack, where the hiker's shoulders can carry the weight, and not on the bottom, where it strains the small of your back. What am I, Danielle Boone? Actually, after three years of scouting now, I guess I am.

Marissa
cable sales manager

And remember, when kids go camping, they're supposed to get dirty, so, on a typical backpacking campout, they're not going to need more than one change of clothes—and that's just for emergencies, or if they run into Mr. Blackwell. Part of the experience is to learn they can actually survive eating food with a little dirt, ash, and . . . what are those? Bugs?

Water, though, is another story. Make sure your kids know that those crystalline mountain streams can contain germs that will make them sick. They should drink only the water they bring or that's okayed for them by an adult.

As for every boy's quest for fire, don't pack matches unless the scoutmaster tells you to. Same goes for knives, hatchets, and basically all the cool stuff your son is going to tell you he absolutely *has* to have.

Girl Scouts generally do less camping, but there's plenty of danger in those cookie drives. All that holiday poundage you wanted to drop? Well, you're right back to square one come February, when you find yourself stuck with a case of Samoas or Thin Mints. If you want to support your daughter's troop and still fit into those new skinny jeans, give the cookies out as hostess gifts when you're invited to dinner parties. Or you can bring a few boxes to a Super Bowl party. If you're not invited to one, host your own and serve them to your husband and his buddies. Nothing goes with beer like chocolate and coconut.

You'll be proud when your little Brownie or Cub Scout starts collecting merit badges, but you'll also have to find a way to put them on their uniform.

*H*annah became a Brownie in second grade, and finally earned a merit badge. I figured it would take just a minute to sew the badge on her sash, but it was backed with this material that made it hard as a rock and nearly impossible to get a needle through. By the time I was finished, *two hours later,* I'd punctured every one of my fingers in a hundred different places.

At the next meeting, I complained to another mom. She said, "Take it to the dry cleaners." I stared at her. "But it wasn't dirty, she hadn't even worn it." "No," she said patiently, "you take it to the dry cleaners and they have this special machine that sews the badges on in about thirty seconds." I felt like a total moron, but I knew as much about scouting as I knew about sewing.

Terry
corporate headhunter

Terry learned a second valuable tip from this other mother: a little bit of club soda mixed with hydrogen peroxide will remove blood stains from just about anything.

No More Pencils, No More Books

Summer vacation is the shortest ten weeks of a kid's life. And the longest of a mom's. It's hot. It's muggy. It's buggy.

And what the heck are you gonna do with those kids for the next two and a half months? Fortunately, there are lots of options for keeping your kid occupied until that joyful day when school resumes.

What the Other Mothers Know

Consider day camp. Depending on your area, however, you may need to have your application in by as early as January. There are a lot of mothers out there with nightmares about bored children stuck in the house all summer, watching reruns.

Many churches offer summer day camp. In addition to Bible study, there are traditional arts and crafts: making trivets out of Popsicle sticks, dreamcatchers, and lanyards, lanyards, lanyards.

And here's your most important consideration when looking for a summer program. It's not about finding a good summer program. It's about finding good summer programs at private schools you want to apply to next year. That way you can commence the sucking-up process early. Many private schools offer summer drama programs, academic enrichment, and sports programs that are open to the general community as well as to their own regular student body. Call the schools in January to get a brochure for their summer programs, and apply early. At the end of the summer, send a nice thank-you note to the principal, full of praise for the wonderful program and how much your child benefited from it. You'll rack up some big points.

Finally, there's the best option of all: sleepaway camp. If, that is, you're sure your child is old enough to handle it. If you're not sure, you can try what this other mother did.

I grew up in Boston, and all my friends and I went to sleepaway camp every summer. Now I live in Los Angeles, and when my husband and I were planning to send our David to sleepaway camp between second and third grade, our friends practically accused us of child abuse. "He's too young!" It got me wondering if maybe it would be too much for David to handle, so, during spring break, we asked him if he wanted to camp out in the backyard with his best friend for a night. "Cool!" he said. We pitched a little tent and the boys made it through the night with no problem. David liked it so much he wanted to do another backyard campout the next night. I figured it was a pretty good test, so we sent in our deposit for sleepaway camp, and off David went that July, for six weeks, and had a great time.

Eleanor
homemaker

Don't forget sleepaway camps for special interests: drama camps, art camps, music camps, "nerd" camps for mathletes and science jocks, space camps, weight-loss camps, and sports camps. (On Catalina Island here in California, there's even a surfing camp for kids. Cowabunga!)

If the tuition at most sleepaway camps is out of your range, contact the Boy and Girl Scouts about their camping programs, which run anywhere from one to eight weeks, and are less expensive than privately owned camps. Over half of all camps offer some level of financial assistance; in addition, there are numerous sources for private funding—churches, community groups, charitable organizations—that can make many youngsters' dream of summer camp a reality.

For those of you who worry how homesick a camper can become, we offer the story of an eleven-year-old attending camp for the first time. As Deron was packing his duffel bag, he vowed to his parents that he would make his counselors' life a living hell. When they anxiously related this to another mother of their acquaintance, she told them to trust the professionals at camp, who'd assured them they'd dealt with exactly this type of situation many times before. "If they can't handle your kid and he doesn't belong there, you'll be the first to know. But stop worrying, because they'll handle him."

After feigning illness the first few days, Deron eventually got into the camp spirit. Here's what his dad, Larry, e-mailed to relatives to update them on Deron's progress:

11-Year-Old Seen Having Good Time at Camp—
Allegedly Participates in Canoeing and Color War

Ann Arbor, MI—Sources tell this reporter that Deron Montgomery, denied medical leave last week after a test for bubonic plague proved negative, was spotted laughing in the canteen with his cousin Ben. But, as the sources of these hopeful reports were all camp employees, verification is sought from Cousin Ben, whose mom has now left a message for him to call her with an eyewitness account.

Other reports indicate that Deron's letters home have ceased to contain non-grammatical threats and vague hitchhiking plans; it has even been rumored that he has made statements regarding his return to camp next summer.

Confirmation cannot be made until Parents Day next weekend.

Larry
orthopedist

Immediately after Larry's mom read this, she faxed everyone a copy of the letter Larry had written her thirty-eight years earlier, when he went to camp for the first time, which began, "Dear Mom and Dad, this place stinks and I hate everybody here!"

Of course, if you want to save yourself a great deal of money and considerable worry, you might try convincing your children's grandparents that they should spend the whole summer with them. At their house.

MORE OTHER MOTHERS' TIPS

- Whatever sport your kid plays, mark his ball and gear by painting his initials on it with nail polish—the darker the better (your perfect excuse for blowing eighteen bucks on Chanel's vixenish Vamp nail polish).
- If you find yourself racing to get to all your kid's activities, hire a trustworthy student to do the driving.
- If you have a housekeeper who does not know how to drive, get her lessons.
- Always keep large- and medium-size thermal bags in your trunk, for transporting cold or frozen items to practices or games.
- Even if you MapQuest destinations in advance, keep local maps or other guides in your car at all times, in case you get lost driving to playdates or away games.
- If you're a single mom, involving your child in soccer or Little League can be a good way for him to develop a sustained, ongoing relationship with an adult male figure.
- If you want your kid's athletic skills strengthened, hire a local high school or college star or assistant coach for private lessons.
- If neither you nor Dad can make the commitment to coach, be the team statistician; you'll learn the game, and you get to sit down the whole time.
- As soon as the season starts, buy a case of drinks for your Snack Day turn; it tends to come around when you least remember it.

- Buy the smallest-size snacks and drinks you can; too often the kids don't finish them, or else they throw them away.
- When it's your turn for Snack Day, bring at least two Hefty trash-can liners for garbage collection.
- Team Moms: bring an e-mail sign-up sheet to the first practice.
- Lining the fields on game morning is easy; recommend this one for your husband if he's not Mr. Jock.
- Putting up/taking down the soccer net is another easy dad chore. (If he balks, remind him that it takes a lot less time than schlepping to the grocery store for all those snacks and drinks.)
- Get your child her own water bottle, so she won't need to find a drinking fountain or borrow from someone else; put her initials on it with nail polish.
- Many art galleries and museums offer private classes on Saturdays; if yours doesn't, ask their community liaison to refer you to instructors in the area.
- Sharing summer child-care: find another family (or two) on the block and hire a neighborhood teenager to keep the kids busy and entertained.
- If your child doesn't know how to swim, enroll him in lessons with a certified instructor so he'll hate her instead of you for making him put his face in the water.

IT'S IN THE BAG

- A scarf and gloves for cold-weather practices and games
- Reading material (if you don't already know the rules of whatever game your child is playing, now would be a good time to learn)
- Thermos filled with hot cocoa or coffee
- Baby wipes
- Toilet paper (when you visit the inside of a municipal-park restroom, you'll understand why)
- Small first-aid kit
- ChapStick
- Elastic holders to keep your daughter's hair out of her face
- Elastic holders to keep your son's hair out of his face
- Granola bars (nut-free)
- Change for vending machines
- Sunglasses
- Sunblock and insect repellent (sometimes they're combined in one product)
- Battery-operated mini-fan
- Needle and thread, Stitch Witchery, and double-sided scotch or toupée tape for costume repair

IT'S IN THE TRUNK

- Portable folding chairs, for sitting at games
- Cushions for hard bleacher seats
- Picnic blanket
- Bottled water
- Sun hat
- Umbrella
- Towels
- A case of soft drinks for the Snack Day that sneaked up on you
- A case of granola bars for that same reason (nut-free)

8

"It's My Party"

(But Somehow Mom Always Has to Clean Up)

Having parties is a social activity that is unique to the human species. Can you imagine a chimpanzee mom inviting all the jungle's young over to celebrate little Ooka's birthday with bananas, grub worms, and some pin-the-tail-on-the-wildebeest? (Who knows, perhaps that *is* what chimpanzees do; it only looks to us like they're picking lice off each other.)

For little girls . . . well, there's a reason why we start clamoring for tea sets before we can walk.

But all kids, girls and boys, must learn the importance of manners, social poise, and being comfortable in groups, so now is the time to start learning how to schmooze.

In this chapter, we share with you some observations and advice on dealing with various social situations, settings, issues, and questions of etiquette, spanning birth through sixth grade. (Yes, birth. If it were up to Hallmark, babies would be given a week to write Mom a thank-you note for bringing them into the world.)

Oh, Behave!

All mothers are proud of their children. Before the delivery-room nurse has finished weighing them, they have become the center of their parents' world. However, that doesn't mean your children are the center of everybody *else's* world.

Back in the old days, most parents understood that when they took their child to a social or public gathering, and the little darling began to scream, it was their job to attend to the problem. Yet, how many of us have been to a wedding, baptism, bar mitzvah, etc., and had to listen to some kid shriek while the parents did absolutely nada? After a while, even God starts giving them dirty looks.

What the Other Mothers Know

Be considerate to all by anticipating that a little one will grow antsy and testy, and take an aisle seat in the back of the room, where you can quickly, quietly slip out if your child starts to get fussy (not to mention, your husband). Not to go all Miss Manners on you, but when it comes to any formal social gathering, etiquette dictates that unless the invitation specifically states, "Mr. and Mrs. So-and-so and Family," your cherub is *not* invited.

Some people assume that if their hosts are especially close friends, they'll be perfectly happy with your children there. Don't. Even if the hostess or bride-to-be is your oldest, bestest friend, tell her a week or two before the wedding that you've either found a sitter, or that you're going to come alone while your husband stays home with the baby. If she insists you bring your child, then go ahead and let the teething toys fall where they may.

I had a friend who brought her two-year-old son to the wedding of a mutual friend. The kid started screaming at the beginning of the exchange of vows and didn't stop. (Why the parents didn't take the kid outside, I don't know.) The bride and groom had hired a videographer, and the little boy completely drowned out their voices. So, when I had a child several years later and was invited to a cousin's wedding, my husband and I rented a room in the hotel where the reception was held. I was still nursing, and it gave me a quiet, clean, comfortable place to be with Alexa, and my husband and I took turns staying with her.

Sheila

contractor

Most of the better hotels have lists of bonded babysitters; contact the concierge in advance to arrange for one. Have the sitter stay in the room with your child, and keep your cell phone on vibrate during the ceremony or the party so you can duck out when called. A great way to keep bigger kids corralled during a wedding or other event is to set aside a table for them and hire a babysitter to watch them; figure one sitter for four to five children, depending on their ages. The ceremony won't be disrupted, and the parents can party in peace.

And no matter how you feel about nursing, *please* don't do it publicly at a wedding or other formal social gathering. There is always a ladies' lounge or anteroom where you can go to nurse your baby. At a wedding, the guests' attention should be focused on the bride's breasts, not yours.

The Fun Never Ends

In elementary school, there's some sort of party just about every month: Halloween, Thanksgiving, Christmas, Hanukkah, Valentine's Day, Easter, Purim, Junior Olympics, End of the Year, and we're convinced that somewhere out there is a school that has a party for Daylight Savings Time. Honestly, it's amazing that kids ever learn the alphabet with all this partying going on. Then again, if you read their Instant Messages, maybe they haven't.

As always, it's the moms who are expected to provide the goodies for these galas.

What the Other Mothers Know

When you are asked to contribute foods for a classroom party, ask your child's teacher if she has a policy on sugared products; some teachers discourage items containing refined sugar. Also inquire about bringing foods containing peanuts; many schools now prohibit them on campus, because of food allergies. But if there's no time to find out, you can always fall back on the default snack: nut-free granola bars and raisins.

If you're asked to prepare a special dish, cook and freeze it in advance, then thaw it the morning of the party. Most schools have a microwave in the cafeteria or faculty lounge, for reheating.

When your child's birthday falls during the week, you might want to let him celebrate it with his classmates, even though he's having a "real" party on the weekend. Of course, this means you'll have to lug in a cake, paper plates, plastic forks, and a long, sharp bread knife that every boy in class will make a grab for.

When Alex was in second grade, I ordered a quarter-sheet SpongeBob SquarePants cake from the bakery and brought it to school, along with candles, paper plates, plastic utensils, and napkins—a lot to juggle. Just when I got about four feet from the classroom door, a kid came tearing out of another class and ran smack into me. The cake flew out of my hands, flipped over, and landed on the floor upside-down. It was completely ruined. The next year, I hit on the solution to the eternal cake question: cupcakes!

Ellen
registered nurse

Cupcakes rule. You only have to bring one candle; and you won't need anything other than wet wipes and something to scrape the icing off the desks. Either buy the cupcakes the day of the party, or, better, have your child help you bake and ice them the night before. (An even better way to go is mini-cupcakes, because the simple fact is, kids *never* eat the cake. They'll take one bite, then run off to play. If you don't want to waste food or money, go with the minis.)

Some teachers balk at allowing more than one student birthday party per week. If you're so unfortunate as to have this kind of wet blanket educating your party animal, try doing what this clever mom did:

*D*arby's third-grade teacher was really down on classroom birthday parties. I didn't want to push it too hard and risk her resenting me and taking it out on Darby, so I thought of this compromise: I suggested that once each month there be one birthday party for all the kids born in that month. I also volunteered to coordinate with the other parents in advance, and assign one parent to handle each month; the teacher wouldn't have to lift a finger. She totally went for it! It was a huge success.

Sharon

insurance adjustor

Regardless of the occasion, never bring popcorn to a class party. Three-quarters of it ends up on the floor, and with so many schools cutting back on janitorial help, it's the teachers who get stuck with the sweeping up. They do not appreciate this. Nor do they appreciate sprinkles, jimmies, confetti, glitter, sequins, tinsel, or pretend fairy dust.

Be aware that many elementary schools, private or public, have a party policy for the younger kids, from kindergarten up through second or third grade: if you invite one child from the class, you should invite *all* the children.

*I*n first grade, my daughter's class had twenty-seven kids. There was no way I could invite all of them to a party at our house, especially since there were kids from the neighborhood and Sunday school she also wanted to invite. Besides that, Karen didn't *like* all the kids in her class, especially the boys. What was I supposed to do? Deny my child a birthday party? Then a friend (a mother of four) suggested I have two parties: one at school, and the other at home.

> *Marcy*
> *computer consultant*

Brilliant. The party at school isn't really a party anyway so much as it is an opportunity for the kids to get a quick sugar rush and sing "Happy Birthday." Schlepping a couple dozen cupcakes to school isn't exactly asking you to host a state dinner, nor is it expensive. For the "real" party that weekend, invite the kids who don't go to school with your child, plus those from her class she really likes.

Another way to avoid having to host your kid's party at a convention center is to invite only the girls from the class if you have a daughter, and only the boys from the class if you have a son. It isn't until fifth grade or so that girls and boys come even close to getting along without screaming "Aaarrrggggghhh, cooties" anyway, so you can usually feel comfortable about restricting the guest list to your child's gender without hurting anyone's feelings.

Kids Just Wanna Have Fun

We all want our children's birthday parties to be special, happy occasions that they'll treasure for life. But too often, parents end up trying to outdo each other with Bigger, Newer, Fancier, and Costlier.

What the Other Mothers Know

Typically, children are perfectly happy with some games, maybe some entertainment (although it's not absolutely necessary), being someplace comfortable they can run around and scream in, and chowing down on kid-type food such as pizza and hot dogs.

Anyone who tells you that you must have a party planner is probably a party planner herself, looking for business. Unless it's for a momentous, more formal occasion, such as a bar/bat mitzvah, a *quinceañera,* or a sweet sixteen, you don't need floral arrangements, Havilland china, or Baccarat crystal, either.

*T*here's no need to hire an entertainer to make a little girl's party special, because they all love tea parties and dressing up. Ask the guests to come wearing Mom's or Grandma's old finery; or you can go to secondhand stores or yard sales and load up on feather boas, long scarves, big hats, opera-length strands of fake pearls, rhinestone earrings, etc., which your daughter and her guests can help themselves to, and which can also be used later on for Halloween costumes or school plays.

If the number of guests is greater than the number of cups in your child's tea set, borrow from a friend or buy an additional set (sterilize them in the dishwasher). Or get an inexpensive acrylic punch set that can do double duty during the summer when you entertain grown-ups—with grown-up rum in the punch.

Another great girlie party is a fashion show. Buy some cheap cosmetics from the drugstore. Open the dress-up trunk and let them put together their outfits. Help them do their hair and makeup. Play some good runway music, and you supply haute couture commentary as the little ladies strut their stuff.

Carina
public defender

Here are some additional tips for hosting a successful party:

- Keep it simple! Moon Bounces? Sure, if you can afford one; kids love them, even though we've never seen one that looked dirty—which, of course, might be exactly why kids love them.
- Cheap entertainment? You can't get cheaper than making the guests provide the entertainment themselves. In advance, write a little play-let based on a nursery tale, like *Little Red Riding Hood* or *The Three Little Pigs;* buy hand puppets appropriate for the story. At the party, ask the kids to decorate a big cardboard box as a puppet-theater stage. Then, you narrate the story as groups of children get behind the "theater" to act it out.
- Party food? Go for plain cheese pizza, hot dogs, hamburgers, chips, and any liquid that's carbonated.
- Do kids need a parade of Disney-clad entertainers to have a good time? Well, we can promise you one thing: your child will *not* end up on a shrink's couch because you didn't hire that Shrek impersonator for his eighth-birthday party.

If you have a pool, you have built-in entertainment.

*I*t was only a week before Jack's seventh-birthday party, and I was desperate to hire an entertainer. But the "Party-saurus" and the "Bob the Builder" rip-off guy seemed pretty lame, especially for the money they wanted. Then it occurred to me: my neighbor's teenage son is a big, strapping kid, a total jock who all the kids idolize, *and* he's a certified Red Cross lifeguard. So I hired him for less than half the money a professional entertainer would have cost, to spend the afternoon letting ten seven-year-old boys roughhouse with him in the pool and chase him around the yard.

It was the best $50 I ever spent: they had a ball; it really meant something to my neighbor's son. And as his mom told me later, after he returned home and collapsed, it was probably the best contraceptive you could ever give a teenage boy.

Judith
stay-at-home mom

And don't sweat the party décor; younger kids have precious little interest in it. Martha Stewart might fret if the pink in the Barbie paper cups doesn't match the balloons, but you should save your artistic flair for when your daughter gets married. You're going to need it when she decides the green of the bridesmaids' gowns' sashes *has* to match the garnish on the salmon croquettes.

A Favor You Can't Refuse

Party favors are certainly not necessary, but they're a nice way to say thank-you to your guests, and they don't have to be fancy or pricey, either. Many party stores, crafts stores, and hobby stores carry all sorts of inexpensive items you can drop into a sack, and kids will treasure them as if they were lifetime passes to Disneyland . . . for about three minutes. Then whatever you put into their swag bags, you'll be picking up from the patio anyway.

Our friend Harriet maintains that piñatas are the leading cause of heart attacks among Southwestern U.S. parents under forty-five. How else do you react when you see a six-year-old boy swinging an aluminum bat around a group of other six-year-olds—blindfolded? Harriet also offers this advice for gringo moms and dads:

> *M*y son Danny begged for a piñata for his birthday party, and after what seemed like hours of watching a dozen kids take a shot at it, my husband took a turn and split the piñata wide open. The kids all screamed and started scrambling over one another to grab the candy. Except . . . there was no candy. Look, I'm a Jewish girl originally from Brooklyn. How was I supposed to know that when you buy a piñata, *you* are the one who supplies the candy? Did it come with instructions? Nooooo. My husband and I yelled, "Time for cake and ice cream!" For years afterwards, whenever Danny saw a piñata at a party, he'd break out in a cold sweat.
>
> *Harriet*
> *artists' manager*

Where's the Party?

Many parents now throw kids' parties outside the home. Laseriums, paint-ball fields, beading and crafts stores, children's theaters, ice skating, roller skating, rock climbing, ceramics stores—these are all fun and exciting venues for a party, depending upon your child's age and interests.

What the Other Mothers Know

But there are other considerations to bear in mind: your guests' *parents'* age and interests.

Last year we attended a party twenty-five miles away. It was one of those party "studios": you tell them what sort of theme your kid is into, and they do it. While our daughter was having a blast, my husband and I were forty-five minutes away from the house; if we drove home, we'd just have to turn around and come right back, so there we were, stuck in a strip mall in some suburb we'd never even heard of before. When it was time for Deirdre's party, she asked to have it at the party studio. Before I sent out the invitations, I Googled the zip code for that area and put together a list of nearby movie theaters, bookstores, and restaurants for the parents to hang out in while they waited for the kids' good times to stop rolling.

Allison

designer

Don't oblige your guests (or their parents) to drive a significant distance unless it's for a theme or activity that is genuinely unique and special. And with gas now the price of platinum, why make anyone spend any more money? (Hey, the less money they spend on gas, the more money they have for your kid's gifts!)

Hey, Let Dad Share in the Fun!

We don't know how or why it happened, but sometime in the last few years it suddenly became Mom's sole responsibility to accompany her young one to birthday parties. Let's work up a quick tally, shall we? Your son's in third grade, and there are at least twenty-four other kids in his class. Even if your little guy gets invited only to the other boys' parties, that's at least twelve parties per school year that you'll have to attend. And that's just third grade. It's one thing for a mother to attend a My Little Pony party with her daughter and stick a plastic Rarity the Unicorn horn on her forehead, but should we females really have to suffer through Roboraptor and Spiderman parties?

What the Other Mothers Know

You've got to find a way to get Dad to step up to the plate—the paper plate, that is. You can always try the old "You could make some good business contacts with the other dads, honey" ruse. But if that doesn't work, appeal to every man's weakness:

> When Tommy was little and the Chuck E. Cheese's commercials came on TV, he'd always start clamoring to go. And I'd say, "Mommy would love to take you, but I don't know where one is." Then all the boys in Tommy's kindergarten class started having their birthday parties there. At the end of the first one, I thought I'd gone deaf; after the second, I was ready to commit hara-kiri. The next time there was a party at Chuck E. Cheese's, I

decided it was *Bill's* turn to take Tommy. "Oh, it's a cute place," I said cheerily. "It's all over in a couple of hours. And . . . they serve beer." When Bill brought Tommy home that afternoon, he looked like a shell-shock victim from the Second World War. He stared at me and moaned, "How could you *do* that to me? And all they had was *light* beer!"

Anne

internist

And for you single mothers who turn ashen at the thought of one more Saturday with some stupid, red-nosed clown (kids or no, we've all had a Saturday like that, haven't we, girls?), ask a childless friend to take your place. For the parent stand-in, it'll be a novelty, spending a few hours with a roomful of kids. Well, once, at least. So if you have no family in the area but lots of gal and guy pals who have not been blessed, we encourage you to turn to them for a respite when you're stricken with birthday-party burnout.

The Gifts You Keep on Giving

We've been waiting to see this on some kid's chest for years: "I Got Carter a Game Boy and All He Gave Me for *My* Birthday Was This Stupid T-Shirt."

Gift competition (what Freud might have called presents envy) seems to have become epidemic. When we were kids, gifts were rarely opened at parties, because our mothers didn't want anyone comparing what the others had bought. The fashion now, however, is to open them after cake has been served.

Don't feel like you have to go into debt to provide a gift for a child's party, especially if your child isn't especially close to the birthday boy or girl. To tell you the truth, most kids would appreciate a piece of gravel so long as it came in a box with gift wrap and a bow on it.

But what if you find yourself in a panic on a Saturday morning an hour before you're expected at a kid's party, and you have absolutely *no* idea what this kid likes?

What the Other Mothers Know

It's easy to buy toys for little kids, because they aren't yet old enough to have developed specific, diverse tastes; all six-month-olds love rattles, or anything else they can drool on. But what do you get for a six-year old-boy you don't know?

I'd seen Jacob at the Little League games, but the only thing I knew about him was that he couldn't hit the backstop, much less the ball. So I was wandering through the toy store, thinking, *Farm animals are probably too baby, but a Megatron Transformer might be a little too violent for his parents . . .* That's when I hit on it: firemen! They're macho, they drive cool trucks that make lots of noise, and they fight fires instead of villains. Whether you're a six-year-old boy or a thirty-six-year-old mom, you've got to love firemen.

Bobbie
human resources director

Excellent.

How about if the birthday boy is a girl? Is a Bratz doll too sexualized and denigrating to women? But would she even want a Super Soaker? A fine compromise that always works with girls is anything artsy-craftsy. There are kits for making costume jewelry, paper flowers, clay sculptures, etc. The finished product is something a girlie girl will love, and a tomboy will enjoy working with her hands and making a mess.

And when you're shopping for a ten-year-old, regardless of gender? At that age, their interests are far more specific; besides, how do you know which DVDs or Nintendo they already have, or if they're even into that stuff?

Give gift certificates or gift cards, preferably from stores that offer a range of items that appeal to a broad range of tastes, such as Blockbuster (they sell both movies and video games) or the big bookstore chains (for books, stationery, DVDs, CDs, etc.). This allows the older kids to choose what they want at a store they like; they won't have to return it because it doesn't fit, or it's the wrong color, or it's not cool enough.

When your children receive a check as a gift, and are old enough to understand what money is and where it comes from (that would be you or Dad), we encourage you to take them to the bank and let them watch how it's deposited, where it goes, and what it does. Anything to do with money is pretty difficult for kids to grasp, because money in and of itself is an abstraction: paper money represents gold (not that any banks even keep that anymore, only at the Federal Reserve), and gold represents the value of what you do. (Deep, huh?) While this won't teach them the value of *earning* money, it will certainly teach them the value of *saving* it, which is every bit as important.

It won't, unfortunately, stop them from begging for more money from you.

The Big Sleep(over)

Kids mature at different rates, but for the most part, they shouldn't have sleepovers until they're seven or eight years old. Actually, we three would've been perfectly happy if our kids hadn't started having them until they were twenty-seven and legally married to the overnight guest.

What the Other Mothers Know

Itty-bitty Jacks and Jillies get the willies when they sleep away from home, and there's nothing less convenient than having to phone Mom and Dad in the middle of the night and tell them their kid is sobbing to come home—except maybe being on the receiving end of the call. This is why God invented playdates. Have your child's friend come home with her after school on Friday, and let her parents pick her up at the end of the evening. It gives the kids plenty of hang time, and the other set of parents the opportunity to go out and see a movie, or have a quiet dinner together—and with a little luck, they'll reciprocate. After a few daytime playdates, the sleepover-er will probably feel comfortable enough at the sleepover-ee's house to make it through the night.

But no matter what their age, never let your kid and his guest watch a scary movie before bedtime. Perhaps horror fare doesn't faze your kid, but your young guest might be more impressionable.

I love horror movies. Vampires, werewolves, ghosts, zombies—if it's scary and done well, I'm there. My son Charlie, who's ten, is also a fan and never gets nightmares.

One Saturday, Charlie's friend Tim slept over, and they watched the original *Night of the Living Dead*, which Charlie has seen a dozen times. About two-thirty that night, my husband and I were wakened by shrieks. Tim, who'd had a nightmare that flesh-eating zombies were coming in through the window, was sweating bullets and reaching for a phone to call his parents' cell. The parents, who are friends of ours, had sent Tim to us and farmed their seven-year-old daughter out to her grandparents, to take their first weekend getaway in years, and I really didn't want to have to interrupt them. I quickly invented the Cannibalistic Humanoid Elimination Weapon (that's CHEW to you). The boys thought my cardboard paper-towel-roll-and-tape zombie zapper was pretty funny, and I eventually got them back to sleep. But I learned my lesson: the last DVD of the evening should always be cartoons!

Daphne

English teacher

Slumber Parties: Threat or Menace?

Why do they call them slumber parties, when no one ever sleeps—especially not the host mom?

Slumber parties aren't usually an issue for boys, because they don't need a whole posse of peers to hang out with. (The paradigm shifts dramatically when they turn sixteen and one of them gains access to a motor vehicle. Then they always seem to have one more friend than seatbelts.)

Girls, however, are different. They tend to have more friends than the typical boy their age, and they want every single girl they've ever met in life to come sleep over and see their new Cinderella Twinkle

Lights Horse-Drawn Pumpkin Carriage. When you have a daughter, figure that, starting when she's nine or ten, you'll be hosting at least one slumber party per annum for her birthday.

*M*y daughter Bailey started begging for a slumber party when she was six years old. I held her off until she was eight, but even then I knew at least half the girls she wanted to invite would never, *ever* make it through an entire night. So, we compromised on a "half-slumber party": the girls would come over in their PJs, eat pizza, watch a DVD, then be picked up by their parents at a very civilized ten thirty or eleven p.m. We did it that way for the next two years, and it was great practice for the real sleepovers.

Ariel
homemaker

Great practice for everything except maybe making prank phone calls to cute boys.

To keep the girls from forming cliques and turning into junior Joan Riverses, dissing each other's nighties, have plenty of group activities ready. Doing hair and makeup is always great for girls; and, it's a great way to get rid of all that makeup you buy that you never use, including the gift-with-purchase samples from department stores. However, under no circumstances allow the beautification ritual to extend to nail polish, unless you want your carpet or coffee table to look like a Jackson Pollock painting. And don't forget to have the girls remove the makeup before they go to sleep (this would be around five thirty a.m.), or your pillowcases will "face" the consequences.

As for coed slumber parties, you'll learn all about those in our sequel . . .

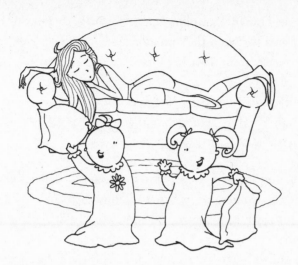

Guess Who's Not Coming to Dinner?

Here's a social conundrum that's absolutely guaranteed to happen to every
parent at least once.

*M*y husband and I were getting ready for a dinner party when
the babysitter I'd arranged for three weeks in advance called at five
forty-five to say she'd just gotten tickets to Hoobastank (it took me
a minute to realize she meant a concert). I started calling other sit-
ters. No luck. It seemed impolite to show up on our hosts' doorstep
with an unannounced guest rug-rat in tow. So, I called our hostess,
explained the situation, and said, "But we hope you'll invite us some

other evening." That gave her the opportunity to say, "Gee, sorry, we'll make it another time," but to my relief, she said, "No problem, just bring Lauren with you."

Jeri
makeup artist

What the Other Mothers Know

Often, you'll find yourself going out to the homes of couples with children, and if they're the same age as yours, you'll both be happy to have your kids occupied. But if you're going to the home of an older or childless couple and you have to bring your child, don't expect your hosts to feed him. And besides, it's embarrassing when your child calls their asparagus vinaigrette "yucky." Feed your child before you leave home. And be sure to grab some kid-friendly DVDs on your way out.

If *you*, however, are the host who now has an unexpected six-year-old guest arriving, and you have a ten-year-old, try hiring your child as a semi-babysitter. She'll feel responsible and important, especially when she gets her bribe—er, payment. And it'll keep your friends' little one from interrupting adult conversation. At least until you get through the main course.

Napkin in the Lapkin

And what if the dinner party is at your "friend" Denny's, Ruby Tuesday's, or Sam Wu's?

No matter how fast the service, kids hate sitting around waiting for food to come with nothing to look at but salt and pepper shakers, so, an establishment with paper placemats and crayons is the way to go. It won't be haute cuisine, but at least you won't have dropped $27 on something your kid just dropped on the floor. Remember, kids don't go to restaurants to chat; they go there to eat. And to drive you nuts.

One evening, for my birthday, we went out with another couple and their children to a nice Chinese restaurant, and my three-year-old, Kevin, was already fidgeting before we were seated. My friend, whose kids were older, nudged a waiter and said, "Bring the little guy a bowl of rice." Sure enough, while we were scanning the menus and chatting, Kevin got his bowl of rice and very happily started eating (when he wasn't trying to fight a duel with the chopsticks). From that night on, I always ordered some small side dish for Kevin the minute we walked into a restaurant.

Brenda
paralegal

The same applies to virtually any kind of cuisine: if it's an Italian restaurant, get your child a side-order of meatballs. If it's a Mexican restaurant, order a cut-up cheese quesadilla. If French, go for some *pommes frites avec sauce tomate très relevée*, but don't worry, they'll stop whining as soon as they see it's fries and ketchup.

If you're obliged to take your child to a more upscale eatery, remember that nouvelle or fusion cuisine is total anathema to most American kids.

They like food that looks like food; at least, food they recognize. Anything puréed is reminiscent of baby food (how insulting). And food that's covered in a sauce will be regarded with suspicion, unless it's spaghetti. So, if the only thing on the menu that she'll eat is chicken, tell the waiter she'd like the chicken Kiev, and hold the Kiev. Most better restaurants don't offer children's menus, but they'll usually accommodate requests for half-orders.

But if a full tummy doesn't help, and your kid is causing your fellow diners to look at you like the Thurston Howells looked at Gilligan, you just might be making the whole thing more complicated than it need be.

*U*ntil Noah was in kindergarten, he'd never been in a restaurant that didn't have a clown logo. When my in-laws visited and took us out to a nice restaurant, he started going absolutely insane: trying to climb into the neighboring banquette, commando-crawling under the table, playing Frisbee with the butter pats—you know, the little-boy drill. Finally, my mother-in-law looked at him and said, "Noah, that's not how you act in a restaurant." Noah just shruggerd. As he was about to make a hat out of Grandpa's napkin, she added, "Noah, do you see Mommy and Daddy acting like that? They have to act differently than they do at home, too." Noah looked at her for a sec, then said, "Oh. Okay." He sat down, put his napkin in his lap, and started drinking his Shirley Temple. Can you believe it? He just didn't know. We'd never thought to tell him that's how you behave in a restaurant.

Mia
exercise instructor

So, if your little party animal is more animal than human, relax. The three greatest forces that will induce your child to stop behaving like a Cro-Magnon in public are parental example, peer pressure, and puberty. All you have to worry about is the first.

MORE OTHER MOTHERS' TIPS

- Take cupcakes to school in a specially designed cupcake carrier: $20, at Linens 'n Things online (www.lnt.com) and Target online (www.target.com); a carrier that holds minis too is available for $20 at www.kitchenkrafts.com.
- When sending e-invites to a party, include a link for MapQuest.
- If money's a factor, think about having an outdoor party at your local park; all you'll need is the cost of a few balloons to decorate the picnic area, and for entertainment . . . they're at a park.
- If the party activities you're planning might make kids' clothes dirty, state so on the invitation.
- Always include directions to, and the phone number of, the venue if you're having a party outside your home.
- If you anticipate any of the children's parents staying for the party, prepare grown-up food for yourself and them (some wine doesn't hurt either).
- When you hold a party at a commercial establishment, make sure to know in advance exactly what you get: does the price include paper goods, a cake, ice cream, food, and soft drinks? Decorations?
- If you're ordering pizza for a party at home, place your order the night before.

- When your child receives gift certificates or cards, keep them in your car so that your child can use them next time you find yourselves at the mall.
- Even if your kid's not a bed-wetter, put a plastic sheet on the mattress, because your kid's friend might be—and remind your husband to wear pajamas.
- Before a sleepover or slumber party in your house, make sure that no one has left an inappropriate DVD in the player or TiVo'ed the Playboy Channel.
- Try not to invite two kids to sleep over; three kids is a recipe for emotional disaster, especially with girls.
- Pack a change of nightgown or jammies; lots of stuff can get spilled on kids during a slumber party.
- When in a restaurant with a toddler, never take a table by the music (he'll try to grab an instrument), or by the front door (he'll try to run out—even if you promise him you're picking up the tab).
- When you have an infant in a carrier seat, turn the restaurant high-chair upside-down so that the wider end is up; you'll find it much easier to contain the carrier.
- If your son orders a Shirley Temple, ask the waiter not to skewer the maraschino cherry with one of those little plastic swords, because boys can turn them into lethal weapons.
- When your pint-size diner leaves an adult-size mess, tip your server generously.
- If your child has the nasty habit of grabbing food off others' plates, try this next time you're at a Chinese restaurant: let him grab something that's been dipped into spicy-hot mustard. That'll cure his rude behavior but good.

IT'S IN THE BAG

- Baby wipes
- Hand-sanitizing lotion
- A gender-neutral birthday card and a $15 Toys "R" Us gift card
- Blank check, for the same purpose
- Cell phone, in case your kid calls you to pick her up early
- Braun Cordless Steam Curling Iron for daughter's last-minute touch-ups
- Pack of tissues for son's last-minute nose-wiping
- Breath mints
- Reading material, pencils, crossword puzzles, and Sudoku for waiting out a party
- Pad and pen for making a thank-you-note list
- Point-and-shoot camera

9

"It's the Most Wonderful Time of the Year"

(Then Why Are We All So Stressed Out That the Dog Is Hiding?)

For children, there's no more magical time of year than the holidays. And for parents, there's nothing more magical than watching their children stand awestruck before that pile of gifts 'neath the tree come Christmas morning, or that basketful of jelly beans and chocolate that the Easter Bunny left on the front porch.

They'd better be, after all that money you just spent.

Now, what do you do when the kid isn't seven any longer and finds out you lied through your teeth about the Tooth Fairy?

What the Other Mothers Know

'Fessing up to your child that the beloved figure you spent years spinning myths about doesn't really exist will send your rapidly beating heart right up into your lying, conniving throat.

What follows is a Christmas classic of Mommy Mea Culpa.

Our daughter, Shea, had Santa figured out when she was in second grade. But our son, Riley, who's seven years younger, was a different story. One day in November, when he was nine, he saw me wrapping gifts to send to relatives, and recognized the paper from the presents "Santa" gave him last year.

"Mom," he said warily, "did you . . . lie to me about Santa?"

Nailed!

I explained that parents want kids to believe in miracles like Santa Claus because it's a good way of helping them understand the true Christmas spirit, of giving, and doing things for others, and Santa is the embodiment of that, blah-blah-blah. I was really worried how Riley would handle this life-changing revelation, but then he leaned over to me and whispered, "Does Shea know?"

Ursula
writer

In other words, it's not that big a deal. No kid has ever gotten on a rooftop with a sniper scope just because he found out his parents love him so much they buy him tons of great stuff every December.

If you have an especially sensitive child, however, and you want to cushion the blow of life without Santa/Easter Bunny/Tooth Fairy, try this: as soon as the news sinks in, shift your disillusioned progeny's attention to all those younger kids who aren't in on The Secret yet. Now it's *his* turn to carry on the tradition and keep the flickering candle of Santa Claus-ness burning in the hearts of those poor clueless tykes.

Nothing perks up a kid more than feeling like an adult . . . an adult who may get to lord it over all those Santa-believin' babies the moment he steps off the school bus. So, if the time has come to tell your child The Truth About Santa, just do what Ursula did and hide that gift wrap right on top of the kitchen table.

Give Till It Hurts. You.

The holidays are fun, but they can be stressful as well, especially with a house full of overnight guests and a big meal to prepare (if the house is full of in-laws, the stress level goes up enough to power your outdoor lights display).

Of course, we all want to give our children the special gifts they've asked for, but sometimes the money isn't there for exactly what they want. Or, as so often happens when an item is immensely popular, even your $100 bribe offer to the loading dock crew at the Toys "R" Us won't work.

And add to that your attempts to inject a little religion into the festivities. Christmas and Easter shouldn't be about gifts or candy but about the religious event each celebrates, and its meaning. But just try to explain the concept of Christ's birth, or rebirth, to a seven-year-old who's still high from half a pound of sugar, doting grandparents, and hours of toy commercials.

What the Other Mothers Know

You can't expect the holidays to rival *Town & Country*'s December issue, but you *can* expect them to be a good deal more fun if you allow your kids to play as active a role in the festivities as they can.

For example, if your little boy is too young to sew a garland of popcorn for the tree, he can still pop the corn in the microwave and dole out the kernels. (By the time he *is* old enough to learn how to sew, he'll protest that it's a "dumb girl's job.")

With a daughter, you can try this:

*O*ne Christmas, when my daughter Kylie was nine or ten, she really wanted to buy her best friend the $20 Evergreen Velvet dress for her American Girl Molly doll. But Kylie only had $13 in her piggy bank. I saw a good opportunity to teach her the value of money, get into the Christmas spirit, and take some of the workload off me. If she'd help sweep up the pine needles all over the living-room floor and mix cookie batter, I'd cover the $7 difference. Three-fifty an hour is a pretty decent wage for a kid, especially when she's getting paid for something that turned out to be fun.

Renee
bookstore owner

When you have very delicate or valuable tree ornaments, hide those from the littler kids and let them put up the less-fragile ones first. Ornaments made of wood, resin, or cloth are best. Soon enough the kiddies will be distracted by some other activity, and you and your husband can move in to finish the job with Great-grandma's precious handblown crystal angels. When the holiday is over, pack the fancy ornaments separately and mark them, so you don't inadvertently hand them to the youngsters next Christmas.

Because ornament hooks usually come in a box or a bag, they wind up getting hooked together (uh, they're hooks), so they're difficult for kids to get out without spilling them all over the place. Pre-hook your ornaments, and store them the same way when you take down the tree; that way the hooks won't wind up on the floor and lie in wait for your vacuum cleaner.

What goes under the tree is always an issue, but *how* it goes under the tree is, too.

*W*hen the kids were little, Doug and I placed the Christmas gifts from out-of-state relatives under the tree a week or so before Christmas, to make it look festive. Then, on Christmas Eve, after the kids went to sleep, we'd put out the presents Santa had brought. On Christmas morning, the kids ran in and tore open the cool Santa gifts that were on top of the pile, leaving their grandparents' and Aunt Trudy's less-cool gifts for last. Worse still, the kids had to sit there for half an hour and watch Doug and me open our gifts to each other. For the kids, it was like going to a movie where all the good scenes are in the first few minutes. Next year, we figured we should build to a climax Christmas morning: we placed some of the Santa gifts we knew they'd love near the base of the tree and saved some of the best for last.

Laurie
computer consultant

And here's a tip that'll save you from being the only one who has to work on Christmas morning: on Christmas Eve, put together some sort of breakfast casserole that can sit in the fridge overnight. When the kids wake up the next morning, pop the casserole into the oven, and breakfast will be ready by the time the gift opening is done. (See chapter 10 for a Christmas morning recipe.)

Hanukkah, O Hanukkah

The month of December can be a tough time for kids who aren't Christian, no matter what their religious background. Christmas is so popular that sometimes even Jewish people tend to forget that the season includes another major holiday: Hanukkah.

When Donna was pregnant with Georgi, a sermon given by her rabbi shortly before the holidays made a deep impression on her; she's followed his sage advice through the years:

The rabbi said it's really hard for Jewish kids during the holidays, because Christmas is everywhere you look—pretty much starting the day after Thanksgiving. He was afraid all this was leaving Hanukkah with very little attention or identity, so, he encouraged us to make Hanukkah as festive as possible, and be sure our kids understood what the holiday meant, no matter how young they were.

So, starting when my daughter was barely a year old, I gave her a gift every night for eight nights (and still do). We'd decorate the house like crazy: blue and silver tinsel everywhere, a menorah in the dining room and one in the front window—we even hung blue garlands on our potted plants. We also have a big party every year, where each kid gets to light one candle. And last Hanukkah we made 140 latkes. The house smelled like a NASCAR time trial for a week, but the latkes were delicious and gone in a flash.

Wherever we are, even on a winter vacation, we light the menorah (a small one, for traveling). Georgi identifies with it as *her* holiday, probably because we've made an effort to put some "ha" in Hanukkah.

Donna

Deck the Halls with Boughs of Challah

When we were interviewing our friends, colleagues, relatives, and acquaintances for material for this book, one issue that came up again and again when discussing the holidays was what to do when one parent is Christian and the other Jewish. This is a question that holds special significance for Ilene and Michele, because we're Jewish but are married to a Catholic and a Protestant, respectively.

What the Other Mothers Know

How—and indeed, whether—to celebrate the holidays is a very important issue in many mixed families, and it can be a complicated one. Here are our stories and the experiences of another friend, which might be helpful to new moms who may someday face this situation themselves.

*B*ecause neither Ben nor I have ever been religious ourselves, we never made religion an issue in our marriage. But Ben and I sincerely believe that any excuse for a party, any excuse for a celebration, any excuse for friends and family to get together and have a good time is worthy. I think our daughter, Nikka, views religion as a sort of a cuisine: she sees the Italian Catholic side as all about meatballs and lasagna, and the Jewish side—matzo balls and brisket.

Ilene

*W*hat Andy and I have done since our kids were big enough to use tinsel for dental floss is celebrate both: we have a tree (with no religious ornaments), latkes, a menorah, and exchange gifts for Christmas and each night of Hanukkah. When Marc was little, a relative asked how he'd know he was Jewish if we had Christmas. I said, "He'll know by going to Hebrew school, and by becoming a bar mitzvah. And if that fails, the first time he sees a foreskin in a locker room full of gentiles I'm reasonably confident that he'll catch on." He did become a bar mitzvah, and our daughter, Abby, a bat mitzvah.

Michele

Our friend Becka added an extra ecumenical twist to the resolution of her holiday dilemma:

We have a mixed family, although my husband, Dave, is not of strong faith. We decided that if we had kids, they'd be raised Jewish. I had no problem with having a Christmas tree, until Matt was born. Then the Great Tree Debate started. Dave begged to keep the tree, but I kept saying, "We're sending mixed messages if we do that." Anyway, we kept the tree, minus any religious symbols. So, instead of a star or an angel on top of the tree, we just got a snowflake-shaped ornament, took out the little metal hookie thing, and stuck it upside-down on the tip-top of the tree. Ta-da!

Every year since, who do you think is always the first person to arrive for our tree-trimming party? My Jewish mom. And she'd probably be happy to come over and decorate yours too.

Becka
high-school teacher

Holidays are supposed to be fun, so why isn't it okay to celebrate the secular aspects of them? After all, you don't have to be Irish to wear green and have a pint o' Guinness on Saint Patrick's Day.

By the same token, all you Christians, Muslims, and Buddhists who want to celebrate Hanukkah? Feel free. The colors are blue, white, and silver; there are eight nights of exchanging gifts and lighting candles; and you put sour cream or applesauce on your latkes (those are potato pancakes). Enjoy.

Boo!

Next to Christmas Eve, Halloween is the biggest night on the kid calendar. Think about it: they get to dress up, terrorize children younger than they are, and even the meanest old man on the block has to give them free candy or risk having his house toilet-papered. (Jewish moms alert: most religious day schools do not allow children to come to class in Halloween costumes; that's saved for Purim.)

There are dozens of costume stores in every metropolitan area, and there are even more outlets on the Internet. Once kids reach the age of four or five, they'll start pestering you for a costume in August, so there's always plenty of lead time.

What the Other Mothers Know

Yet, sometimes even the best-laid plans of mice and moms go wrong . . .

When Jordan was ten, we bought him a really neat pirate costume. Before he left for school, Jordan proudly laid the costume out on his bed. While I was at the office, the cleaning lady put the costume in the wash. That wasn't so bad. But then she put it in the dryer. The plastic belt melted into the fabric, and the nylon fabric was in shreds. We didn't discover the problem until six-thirty p.m. Jordan's friends were coming over any minute to go trick-or-treating, but Jordan was so upset he didn't want to go. I had to come up with something, fast. When I suggested he wear some of my clothes and go in drag, both he *and* my husband vetoed it. So, we put his pants, shirt, and baseball cap on backwards, then added a pair of sunglasses on the back of his head.

And Jordan became . . . Nadroj, the Backwards Boy.

Teresa
administrative assistant

The other mothers also know that selecting an appropriate costume can sometimes be trying, especially with older kids, who love dressing up like crazed, ax-wielding serial killers. But even younger ones can drive you crazy, especially when they're too little to understand why the costume they've selected makes you cringe.

*L*ast year, my son Teddy announced he was going as Death for Halloween. You know, the black hooded cape, a glow-in-the-dark skeleton mask, and a very realistic-looking scythe. I found it a horribly morbid costume for a six-year-old, but when I asked my mother how to talk Teddy out of his shroud, she reminded me that when I was seven, I insisted on dressing up like an Old West dance-hall girl. "So?" I asked. "Katie," she said, "the phrase 'dance-hall girl' is a euphemism for 'hooker.' It wasn't dancing they were doing in those saloons."

Well, I got my mom's point, but this year, he's going as Nemo.

Kate
homemaker

Besides discovering that her mom had become a big fan of *Deadwood*, Kate learned that, as happens so often when raising children, you have to choose your battles. The whole point of Halloween is to be naughty, in a safe way. So, as long as they're not wearing Freddy Krueger talons to school, lighten up.

Another issue that arises on Halloween the moment your kids walk in the house from their evening of extorting sucrose-laden products from your friends and neighbors is handing their loot over. Sure, they'll cry and whine and plead to take it into their rooms, and swear on their lives they'll eat only two pieces a day, but don't you fall for it. Put each child's candy into a big Ziploc bag, then store the bags where they can't reach them.

Of course, there's no law that says you can't put those candy bags within *your* reach.

If your kid goes ballistic that he can't devour all his treasure in one fell swoop, or, if she gets mad because you made her share her haul with the little brother who didn't get anywhere near as much as she did, remind them that Halloween candy isn't a right, it's a privilege.

*M*y daughter Vickie always came home with more candy than Willy Wonka. There's no way I'd let her pig out on all that stuff, but it was becoming such a battle that I was dubbed the Grinch of Halloween. So, I came up with a candy allotment system: she'd get one piece of candy per day, but if she did something special, like coming home with an A on a test or playing with her little brother, I'd let her reach into the bag for a handful. Thank goodness Vickie's not a better-behaved kid or she'd be the size of a whale.

Stephanie
librarian

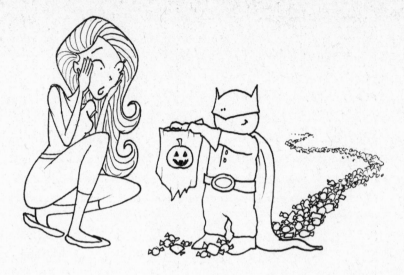

Warning: unless you want to spend Halloween night retracing your child's steps, *never* send a trick-or-treater out with a paper bag. If he drags the bag along the ground, the evening frost or dew will turn the bottom into pulp, and before he knows it he'll have left a trail of miniature Butterfingers and Tootsie Pops all over the neighborhood.

Turkey Day

Thanksgiving is another holiday much beloved by children, even if it doesn't come with presents and candy. And it's even more beloved by husbands, because it combines eating and football.

What the Other Mothers Know

If you're hosting the big dinner, you can get your children involved in many ways, like having them decorate the table. Send them out to the yard to look for the most colorful autumn leaves they can find. Later, when they're tired from all that running around, have them arrange the red, yellow, and golden leaves in a glass vase or bowl—along with the piece of bark and the squirrel-chewed pinecone that will probably come with them. Even if it's not the most gorgeous centerpiece, it kept them out of your hair for a couple hours, right?

And as far as cooking goes, there are several ways to enlist children's aid and make them feel like they're contributing to the Turkey Day festivities. You can ask them to grease baking pans, stir ingredients (in large bowls), and listen for the timer.

Generally, little girls are squeamish about helping to stuff the turkey. It's a chore most of us grown-ups hate too, but for little boys? "Ewwww, gross, Mom! I wanna do it!"

Starting when Ryan was seven, I gave him a pair of small disposable cellophane gloves (available at drugstores, and in bulk from restaurant-supply stores), and placed the turkey breast-up on our butcher block island so that it resembled a patient on an operating table. "Mr. Turkey, the doctor will see you now." Doctor Ryan would put a Fisher-Price stethoscope around his neck, pull on his gloves, and examine the patient. I'd hand him the bowl of stuffing and he'd very carefully shove it inside the cavity.

Remember that little hands should be washed immediately after touching any raw poultry, to avoid salmonella. And make sure you supervise your little doctor closely; one year, we started carving the turkey and found a glove inside.

Dallas

homemaker

Take advantage of this while they're little, because the window of opportunity is open only so long; ask them for help in the kitchen when they're twelve, and they look at you like you just asked them to pay for their own orthodontia.

But there is one potential danger zone in this least stressful of holidays . . . when you have more than two kids, and only one wishbone.

Several Thanksgivings ago, the whole family came to dinner, including my sister and her two kids. The older, Daniel, was about the same age as our son, Harry, so, after dinner, when it came time to pull the wishbone, I was just about to hand it to them when my little niece, Cheryl, set up a howl: she wanted to pull it too. Silly me, for not making two turkeys. I didn't want to leave Cheryl out, but the two boys were getting antsy to snap that turkey bone. I started thinking about how to defuse the situation, and thought about another holiday: all kids love Easter-egg hunts. What if I hid the wishbone somewhere in the living room, and let the kids search for it? Whoever found it got to pull the wishbone with me.

It was Daniel who found it. I told him to talk to the other two kids and come up with a group wish for the three of them. Then we grabbed the wishbone, and sure enough, Daniel won. (If you hold your end of the wishbone lower than your opponent does, you're guaranteed to lose.)

Maria Elena
math teacher

When in doubt, find a way to put kids on the same side—preferably, against an adult. They'll band together like buffalo in a blizzard every time.

Be Mine

What used to be called Saint Valentine's Day still holds heavenly meaning for sweethearts the world over, despite the fact that the Church rescinded the poor guy's sainthood back in the 1960s, as a result of his questionable historical origins.

What the Other Mothers Know

If your son wants to send valentines, let him choose the cards himself. There's nothing more humiliating to a boy than to watch all the girls in his class open his cards and gush over the gooey sentiments his *mom* selected from the rack at the drugstore. Best way to go? The funny kind.

What do you do if your son *doesn't* want to give out valentines but everybody in his class is going to? You don't want him to be left out; at the same time, you don't want to force him to do something that'll make him hurl (Valentine's Day isn't really supposed to be for kids, anyway, but for grown-up lovers).

Here's another mother's Valentine's Day alternative to cards.

$\mathcal{M}$y son Charlie is what you'd call a real boy's boy, and incredibly shy around girls, so he always hated Valentine's Day. By the time he reached fourth grade, he was totally grossed out by the prospect of giving cards with little hearts and flowers on them. I didn't want him to show up empty-handed, and he'd worked himself into such a state that he didn't want to go to school at all. On February 13, I found a solution: Charlie loves chocolate-chip cookies, so, when he came home from school that afternoon, I'd already mixed the batter, and he helped me drop the spoonfuls onto the baking sheets—one cookie for each kid in his class, and one for the teacher. I took the big heart-shaped box of candy my husband had bought me, and put the cookies in that. Charlie got through Valentine's Day without embarrassment; in fact, I think he impressed quite a few girls.

Olivia
interior designer

"You Lied About the Bunny <u>Too</u>, Mommy?"

A child's discovery that the Easter Bunny, too, is fictitious is easier for her to accept once she's learned that Santa Claus is fictitious. (After you've destroyed their innocence by dropping the dime on Santa, they're usually too jaded and cynical to care who brings the jelly beans and the chocolate eggs, just so long as they bring them.)

Which brings us to the most important issue of all: indoor Easter-egg hunts, or outdoor?

What the Other Mothers Know

Outdoors means more hiding places, and less mess in the house.

On the other hand, indoors means fewer grass and mud stains on kids' clothes. Plus, you can go out in your bathrobe at seven a.m. to hide the eggs, instead of having to get dressed and skulk around your dew-drenched forsythia.

But wherever you stow the eggs, the biggest problem you're likely to face comes when you have children of different ages participating: how do you rig it so that the little ones find some before the big kids grab them all?

We have three kids, age four, seven, and ten. And every year, we always have the same problem at Easter: the ten-year-old, Mike, finds most of the eggs; seven-year-old Holly is lucky to get a couple, and little Evan doesn't have a snowball's chance. I hate to see the younger two feel bad on Easter morning, but how do you tell the oldest to not look so hard? It wasn't like he was cheating; he's just older and taller.

My husband, Lou, and I came up with a solution: I had him hide an egg in plain sight, but up in a low-hanging tree branch. Mike spotted it immediately and spent the next ten minutes figuring out how to shake it down or knock it down with a stick. That gave Holly time to find some of the eggs in the usual places (behind a planter, by the mailbox, etc.). And for little Evan, we'd hidden eggs in our bathrobe pockets. That way when he toddled up with his empty basket ready to start whining, we'd put him on our laps, where he'd "accidentally" find the last four eggs.

Thea

physician's assistant

Incidentally, a nice change of pace from dyeing chickens' eggs is . . . dyeing goose eggs. Seriously. Goose eggs are three times the size of hen's eggs, which makes them a whole lot easier for small hands to decorate. Goose eggs are available from January to July; you can order them online or Google a retailer near you.

Passover

If you're not Jewish, you've probably heard of Passover, although you might not know what it's about. After Rosh Hashanah (New Year) and Yom Kippur (the Day of Atonement), the next biggest Jewish holiday is Passover, when we celebrate the ancient Hebrews' flight from Egypt, where—oh, just rent *The Ten Commandments*.

On Passover, instead of fasting like we do on Yom Kippur, we eat. A lot. This dinner is called a Seder. And remember how your mom always told you not to read at the dinner table? We *have* to read at the table, from a little book called a Haggadah, which tells the story of Passover.

Marty and I held a traditional Seder when our kids were six and eight, but the kids couldn't relate to the Maxwell House Haggadah. We wanted something they could understand and really get into, so, we decided to write a kid-appropriate Haggadah. Marty and I wrote the bulk of it in the simplest language possible, then we assigned the Plagues to the kids; there are ten of them, and they're the best part of the story. Each child took five plagues and wrote about it (or dictated to us to write) in his or her own words. It's not only funnier, but it's far more meaningful. The kids enjoy it so much that we update it every year, and it's become almost a time capsule of our family.

Mimi

pharmaceutical sales rep

If you and yours aren't that literarily inclined, you can find family-friendly Haggadahs online. Finding a good kosher wine, however, is another story.

Independence Day

The Fourth of July is another secular holiday that kids love, because what kid doesn't love watching stuff explode? What dad doesn't want to watch a baseball game on TV, followed by some manly barbecuing? And what mom doesn't enjoy the only holiday in which a lot of men actually do the cooking, the plates and silverware can be thrown away, and you can let any fallen food turn into mulch?

And any excuse to buy the red, white, and blue M&Ms is always welcome.

Unfortunately, the Fourth of July is also potentially the most dangerous holiday.

What the Other Mothers Know

Everybody wants to see fireworks on Independence Day, but not in their kid's hands.

The best way to view a fireworks display is to get friendly with someone who has a house on the beach; most coastal cities and seaside communities put on magnificent fireworks displays over the water.

If you're landlocked, become the new best friend of someone who has a view of the local fireworks. It's a heck of a lot nicer than fighting traffic in order to lug a cooler, diaper bag, and a blanket half a mile for the privilege of sitting on a damp football field.

If you can't get to a public fireworks display, and your husband has the impulse to engage in DIY pyrotechnics, buy sparklers. They're legal, and safe (with adult supervision, duh) for getting your rockets' red glare on.

But face it, "legal" and "safe" aren't exactly the two favorite words of most little boys. How do you put on a backyard fireworks display without the fire? Something really cool, but that isn't going to leave little Billy with the nickname Lefty?

*M*y nine-year-old son Cory loves anything that's loud and scary, and every Fourth of July, he begs my husband, Frank, for something sure to make the long weekend a nightmare for me. And the dog. One day, driving home from work, I was listening to a story on National Public Radio, about these guys who figured out that if you drop a Mentos in a two-liter plastic bottle of diet soda, it erupts instantly into Old Faithful. So, I thought maybe that would make the boys happy. It's not dangerous, and it's not fire, but at least it's messy and sticky and really cool to watch. I bought a case of Diet Coke and Mentos. Later, when Cory and Frank were listening wistfully to the distant pop-pop-pops of various neighbors flouting the law, I brought out the stuff and showed them how to set it off. We all had a blast—literally. (My advice: bring plenty of towels.)

Deanne
auto broker

Oh, and if you're friendly with any Brits and you want to see some emotional fireworks, remind them that we won.

Let's Pack Up and Go

Of course, the most daunting holiday of all is the traditional family vacation.

First of all, let's define vacation. Visiting your parents? Not a vacation. Visiting your spouse's parents? A vacation in Hell. Splitting your vacation between your parents and your husband's parents? A vacation in Hell for you *and* your husband.

Vacations are predicated on the notion of leaving your home (Point A) and journeying to some destination that is not your home (Point B). Keeping kids occupied on a train or a plane isn't always the easiest thing to do, but at least you can get out of your seat and walk up and down the aisle with your fussy three-year-old.

That is not, however, feasible when you're traveling by car, because children need to be in a car seat at all times, or, if they're older, seat-belted.

If your butt was squashed into a tiny plastic seat for hours on end, you'd get pretty cranky too.

*P*eter never had problems on short trips, like going to day care or to the store; but when he was twenty-six months old, we drove from Delaware to the Smoky Mountains. Seven hours. He played with one toy for a few minutes, dropped it on the floor, picked up another one . . . half an hour into the trip, he'd tossed all his toys. My husband and I couldn't reach over to pick up what he'd dropped, nor were we about to set a precedent of pulling over to do so. Peter started screaming and screaming. That's when we decided to do something we'd sworn we'd never do when we had kids: install a TV monitor and DVD player in the backseat. Our trip back home wasn't measured in miles but in *Ice Age* (once), *Baby Wordsworth* (three times), and *Elmo's World* (twice). My motto? "Peace, at any price."

Lisa
industrial chemist

What the Other Mothers Know

We're not advocating that you put on a DVD every time a kid cries during a road trip. Hardly. Most kids, even toddlers, watch far more television than they should anyway.

But when you're traveling? Anything goes, because you simply cannot expect regular behavior from a kid in a car. There are only so many diversions you can offer in a moving vehicle: singing songs, toys, and food—the same methods that mothers have used ever since Henry Ford invented the Model T, and he and Mrs. Ford took baby Edsel on his first trip to Grandma's house. The TV/DVD-player option on most new cars is pricey; if you can't afford that, another option is bringing a portable DVD player or computer.

*F*or car trips, we pack Justin's backpack with his favorite toys and books; he keeps that in the backseat with him. But mostly that's just for security; nothing occupies his time better than a new toy or book, so that's why we also bring a stash of small new toys and books that we dole out to him throughout the trip. (You can get some real finds at the dollar store.) We've been doing this since he was around two and a half. If he behaves, then each time we stop for gas or food, he gets to pick out a treat from the stash for the next leg of the journey. Now that he's four, he's traveled thousands of miles with us with a bare minimum of whining.

Gail

accountant

Bring everything you can to keep your child entertained, and don't worry about it spoiling him or her. It won't. As soon as vacation time's over and you're all back at home, it's back to business. When you go on vacation, you don't have to go to work or get up at a particular time; shouldn't your child be given the same latitude?

Though hotels are expensive, don't rule out big-city vacations with kids. You never run out of things to do, and in the summer, lots of it is free (concerts and theater in the park, seeing national monuments, etc.).

Try vacationing in New York City with your child. For kids who don't live in a multicultural community, it's a real treat to eat all the different foods, hear the different music, see the different people on the streets. And the only thing cooler than riding a train is riding one that goes underground. Other good big-city destinations for children are Washington, DC, Boston, Philadelphia, Chicago, and San Francisco. (If you take your children to San Francisco, by all means see Chinatown and ride the cable cars. But whatever you do, do *not* miss the Alcatraz tour. There's nothing better for making kids behave.)

Going on a cruise is an excellent family vacation. Costs are controlled (if you stay away from the roulette wheel and keep your shore excursions to a minimum), and there's tons to do. All the cruise lines have kids' and teens' programs, and offer optional private babysitting after hours. Some of the cabins can hold up to four people; and inside cabins in general are very affordable (since you're there with your kids, you don't need a romantic view anyway). We still exchange holiday greetings with a family we met on an Alaskan cruise ten years ago.

Syd
furniture designer

If you're trying to combine a kid-friendly vacation with a parent-friendly vacation, in natural surroundings, check out family camp.

Family camp has existed since the early 1900s, when it became fun and fashionable to do exactly what mankind had just spent half a million years trying to get away from: living outdoors. But it's a great thing to do when the kids are little, because, for starters, it allows them to get a camping-like experience while offering all the conveniences of a resort.

I loved family camp; we went three summers in a row. I could check my kids in and forget all about them for hours at a time. I could go to the crafts room and spend hours crafting a wooden picture frame or sewing an apron, didn't matter. I read my book. I took naps. I went for walks and bike rides without worrying about my kids getting run off the road. It really allowed me to clear my head.

Our camp had care for every age, including infants. (The first time we went, I checked my youngest, Douglas, in there when he was seven months old; I'd just show up to nurse, then go on my merry way.) All of my kids enjoyed it, especially my older son, Jonathan, who loved the fact that college tennis coaches came yearly and would play with him till he dropped.

Overall, it was just the right amount of freedom, combined with just the right amount of supervision; and everything age-appropriate. And there were enough family activities that I never felt guilty about leaving the kids. The rooms are very simple but clean, and easy to deal with. And the food was actually good—definitely not the Swiss steak, Kool-Aid, and Jell-O repasts I remember from camp when I was a kid.

Joyce
attorney

For a fine resource for every sort of family vacation, from white-water rafting in Colorado to camping on the grounds of a French chateau, go to www.familytravelguides.com.

Another Other Mother summertime vacation tip is renting a beach house.

*I*t's definitely more convenient than staying in a hotel, because the kids can make all the noise they want, and you can do your own laundry. Plus, having a kitchen makes it much easier and cheaper for meals. Everyone can be on a different schedule, getting up at different times, eating breakfast whenever they get up. And you don't have to deal with entertaining kids three meals a day at restaurants.

Having the extra room at a house is also good, so that the kids can go watch TV or play in another part of the house and provide some sanity for the adults. If you're looking to save money, you can stay a few blocks off the beach. But with little kids, I think it's worth it to be as close to the water as possible, especially when they're constantly running back to the house for potty breaks.

Karen
executive assistant

If you can afford a resort vacation, look for one that offers spas and adult activities for you and Dad, and programs to keep the kids occupied and out of your hair, so you can get it cut and styled.

Wherever you go, always make sure that they have programs for whatever age kids you have, so that you can do what you want to do and they can pursue their own interests with their peers. Always check what the minimum age is for the children's programs; at most of them, the kids must be at least four before they can take horseback-riding or skiing lessons.

If your husband balks at a resort vacation or a cruise, consider a dude ranch.

*M*y husband, Felipe, isn't what you'd call the vacation type. It's not because of the money, by any means. Lounging around a pool getting massages is *my* idea of heaven, but it's nowhere near active enough for Felipe. His idea of fun is working in his wood shop, or building a recording studio in the backyard. But then I came across dude ranches online, and checked them out. Horses, hayrides, coyotes, and rattlesnakes sounded about his speed—plus they still had the spa, masseuses, and tennis courts for me and the kids. Felipe had a blast playing cowboy, and so did the kids and I, playing in the pool with a bit of riding and sunset-gazing thrown in. Well, the one thing that wasn't so much fun was that time he made us get up at five a.m. for the chuck-wagon breakfast ride. I'm sorry, but *no* pancakes are that good.

> *Bobbi*
> *pension fund administrator*

Vacationing at an all-inclusive resort for families, such as Club Med, is another excellent way to recharge the batteries of both school-weary children and work-weary parents.

*A*s a single mom, I found Club Med to be a real godsend. I could eat meals with other adults and enjoy grown-up activities like tennis, while my daughter was at the kids' camp all day, making friends and having fun. I could be as busy as I wanted to, or I could just lie on the beach for hours with a book and a piña colada. But no matter what I was doing, I never felt alone, or lonely.

And there were always one or two cute single dads!

Donna

No matter where you go for your vacation, and no matter what you do, the purpose is for you and your family to relax, have fun, and enjoy your surroundings. Notice we said "you." A vacation is time for Mom to cut loose too, so don't waste one precious moment of it by hauling the children into the bathtub every single night, or cooking an elaborate meal. Just because you have kids doesn't mean you can't be as carefree as one yourself, when the occasion permits.

MORE OTHER MOTHERS' TIPS

- Help kids go to sleep on Christmas Eve by establishing a yearly ritual (watch a Christmas movie, read "The Night Before Christmas," then off to bed); it'll save arguing over how late they can stay up.

- When you take an older child out to buy Christmas gifts for her friends, do it in November, so that you can find out what *she* wants for Christmas.

- When you trim the lower branches off the Christmas tree, save them for the kids to make mini-wreaths and other little decorations.

- If you have crawdlers in the house, don't hang tree ornaments or lights within their reach; a table-top tree is the safest way to go.

- Don't insist your tree be perfect; you're not decorating Macy's window. A perfect tree isn't nearly as important as a shared family event.

- Instead of letting tiny tots light Hanukkah candles, let them put Velcro candles on a stuffed, cloth menorah (available at most Judaica stores).

- Little kids love it when you hide the Hanukkah presents. After you light the candles, play "hot or cold" and watch them sniff out those gifts like bloodhounds.

- If you're having a Halloween or Christmas party and kids are attending, don't put candles on buffet, coffee, or side tables, where kids will reach for treats.

- Always use a round-tipped pumpkin knife to carve your jack-o'-lantern.
- Let kids have some delightfully yucky fun by reaching inside the pumpkin and pulling out Jack's brains.
- After scooping out the pumpkin seeds, wash them and bake them, for a tasty and nutritious snack.
- Wait until Halloween to set out your jack-o'-lantern. Putting it out sooner can be an open invitation to local pranksters, leaving you pumpkin-less on the big night.
- Pumpkins are vegetables, and vegetables rot. A jack-o'-lantern's life span is four to five days.
- Ask the other mothers in your neighborhood which are the best trick-or-treating blocks in the neighborhood, and which houses have the best decorations.
- Jewish schools frown upon Valentine's Day cards, so check your school's policy before your kid shows up with conversation hearts for the entire third-grade class.
- When hiding Easter eggs in the house, make a little map of where you put them and spare yourself the stench that accompanies an undiscovered egg.
- Kid-friendly Passover Seder decorations and kits are available in selected stores nationwide, synagogue gift shops, and Judaica stores (we especially like the "My Passover Seder Kit" distributed by Alef Judaica).
- Use fireplace lighters to safely light sparklers.
- When your child starts losing her baby teeth, keep dollar bills on hand to "lend" to the Tooth Fairy; keep the bills by your nightstand so you won't forget before you go to sleep.
- Get a travel agent who specializes in finding fun kid- and family-friendly vacations.

- When you drive to a vacation with a child under six, and if you have room in the car, bring a step stool for the hotel, so he can wash his hands and brush his teeth.
- Always bring any prescription medicines you might need, and over-the-counter basics such as children's aspirin, decongestants, Pepto-Bismol, and Kaopectate along on your trip, especially if you're going to an out-of-the-way spot or to a foreign country.
- When staying in a rental house or hotel, bring safety plugs for the outlets if your kids are little. They're cheap and take only a second to insert.
- If your summer rental has stairs and you have a toddler, bring a gate if the house doesn't already have one.
- When you arrive at a rental house, check the kitchen and bathroom cabinets for any cleaners or other hazards, and rearrange if necessary.
- Whenever possible, get a rental house that has a washer and dryer.
- Find out if towels and sheets are provided or if you need to bring those.
- Going in on a summer rental with another family helps keep the costs down *and* gives your child a built-in companion.
- Kids—and grown-ups—come down with summer colds and other illnesses. If you've planned a special vacation that's costing you bucks deluxe, learn about vacation insurance. (Yes, vacation insurance. Ask your travel agent.)

IT'S IN THE DVD PLAYER

No matter what the holiday, kids (and parents) can always use a little downtime amid the festivities to relax, snuggle, and forget about those pies in the oven.

There are hundreds of holiday DVDs for kids age two through seven, both in animated versions and live action. What we offer below, in calendar order, is a list of our favorite holiday films appropriate for children eight and up; all are available on DVD.

Valentine's Day

The Princess Bride (1987, PG) appeals to both girls and boys, combining a fairy-tale romance with plenty of action, humor, and swordplay; adults will appreciate its sly wit and fine performances. *Lady and the Tramp* (1955, unrated) is a timeless love story, even if the lovers are furry, have tails, and eat spaghetti without a fork. And the retro-screwball romantic comedy *What's Up, Doc?* (1972, PG), with Barbra Streisand and Ryan O'Neal, contains side-splittingly funny physical comedy.

Saint Patrick's Day

Darby O'Gill and the Little People (1959, PG) is hands-down the best leprechaun movie ever made. Even better, girls, it stars the young, radiantly handsome, and hirsute Sean Connery in one of his first film roles. Erin Go Bond! (Never, and we mean *never,* let your kids watch any of the *Leprechaun* film series; the main character, a diabolical leprechaun, is a serial killer. Yes, a serial killer. Hey, we don't make this stuff up.)

Easter

Most of the feature films made about Easter are either boring (*The Greatest* [Longest] *Story Ever Told*), or violent (*The Passion of the Christ*). While *Ben-Hur* (1959, G) stars Charlton Heston as a Judean fighting the Romans, the subplot is the nascent Christian movement, culminating in the Crucifixion. Best of all is *The Robe* (1953, unrated), the first wide-screen film ever, which tells the story of the Crucifixion (from a Roman point of view) and the martyrdom of the early Christians in the Roman Coliseum.

Passover

A Rugrats Passover and *A Rugrats Chanukah* (1991, G) are a treat for young and old. Admittedly, *The Ten Commandments* (1955, G) is a whole lotta ham to serve on Passover, but the parting of the Red Sea still keeps kids on the edge of their seat. (Heston played so many Jewish characters we should've granted him the Right of Return.)

The Fourth of July

There are very few films about the American Revolution, but the best are Disney's *Johnny Tremain* (1957, G), "The Swamp Fox" (a *Wonderful World of Disney* miniseries about the spy Frances Marion), *The Howards of Virginia* (1940, starring Cary Grant, unrated), and *Drums Along the Mohawk* (1939, unrated), directed by John Ford.

Halloween

Except for Christmas, no other holiday has inspired so many movies as Halloween; too bad most of them are R-rated gore-fests. But we have some favorite exceptions: *Love at First Bite* (1979, PG), with George Hamilton as the disco-feverish Dracula in a spoof adults will enjoy too. *Hocus Pocus* (1993, PG) features Bette Midler, Sarah Jessica Parker, and Kathy Najimy as seventeenth-century witches haunting teenagers in modern-day New England. B-movie classic *Abbott & Costello Meet Frankenstein* (1948, unrated) is guaranteed to make kids giggle (they also meet Dracula *and* the Wolf Man, what a bargain). And ultra-campy fun for (much) older kids is *The Rocky Horror Picture Show* (1975, R).

While the following Halloween films' special effects are limited, what they lack in scares they more than make up for with their eerie mood and tone: *Frankenstein* (1931), *Dracula* (1932), *Bride of Frankenstein* (1935), and *The Wolf Man* (1941), all unrated.

Today's kids, accustomed as they are to CGI-laden movies, will find them quaintly but appealingly retro.

Thanksgiving

Everybody loves watching *Miracle on 34th Street* (1948, G) for Christmas, but the first half-hour is all about Thanksgiving and the Macy's parade. *Squanto: A Warrior's Tale* (1994, PG), tells the story of the *Mayflower*'s arrival from a Native American perspective (just don't expect much in the historical accuracy department).

Hanukkah

Oy vey. Thousands of Jewish people in show biz and the best we can come up with is *Eight Crazy Nights,* which isn't even about the holiday (and rated PG-13)? Adam Sandler, however, gloriously redeems his participation in *Nights* with his "Hanukkah Song," appropriate for kids of any age (available for download from various Web sites).

Christmas

We've all seen the classics: *It's a Wonderful Life, White Christmas, A Christmas Story, Miracle on 34th Street,* all 9,287 versions of *A Christmas Carol,* and the perennial children's television favorite, "A Charlie Brown Christmas" (1965, G). Here are several family-friendly films you might not immediately associate with Christmas, but which include memorable holiday sequences: *Heidi* (1937), *Meet Me in St. Louis* (1944), *O. Henry's Full House* (1952), and *Babes in Toyland* (1961), all unrated.

10

"Yummy, Yummy, Yummy, I Got Love in My Tummy"

(Now You Gotta Find a Way to Get It on the Table)

Just as we grow up in all different kinds of houses and families, we grow up with all different kinds of cuisine.

There's nothing like food to evoke memories, with its smell, texture, and taste. Like Marcel Proust and his madeleine cookies, sometimes all we need is a faint aroma to bring our entire childhood back to us. (Of course, that doesn't mean you have to launch into a thousand-page book about it, like he did.) You smell onions frying and suddenly you can see your mom making chili from scratch, smiling at you from across the kitchen while you sat at the table, trying to muddle through long division or the Missouri Compromise.

As your children grow, they will begin to associate certain foods with you and your home together; someday, so will your grandchildren (hard to imagine while their parent is still in diapers).

But what happens if you're not a good cook?

I love to eat, but I just don't get into cooking the way some people do. But we always have a ton of food in our house, because our son Eric is a football player. He's only in tenth grade but is already six foot two, and weighs over two hundred pounds, so he's constantly feeding the machine. My husband and I usually don't get home till seven on week-nights, so, during the school year, we order in or get takeout on the way home—good stuff, though, not fast-food junk.

Then Eric started dating a girl whose mother is a fantastic, world-class cook; she made us a *bûche de Noël* for Christmas, which, if you know anything about food, tells you she knows her stuff. So, Eric started getting on my case to cook like Janie's mom. Finally, I said, "Look Eric, I don't know how to cook. I'm sorry." He looked at me as if I were a total idiot, rolled his eyes, and said in this very patient voice, "*Mom.* Just go to Janie's house, sit at her kitchen table, and watch what her mom does."

Candace
software developer

Candace, of course, did not decide to spend every waking hour watching her son's girlfriend's mother whip up bird's-nest soup or *paella Catalán*. What she did do was start putting her store-bought entrées and side dishes on serving platters, so her family could sit down together and eat. She suspected rightly that what her son was really looking for had less to do with his refined palate and more with his yearning for a "family moment."

What the Other Mothers Know

The fact is, the food at everyone else's house *always* tastes better than yours.

Nicky's skinny as a stick. Maybe it's genetics, but I think it has more to do with his being the world's pickiest eater. I know, probably every mother in the world says that her kid is the worst. He's so fussy that we started calling him Fin-Nicky when he was two.

One morning, when Nicky was in third or fourth grade, I went to pick him up from a sleepover. When he got inside the car, I was amazed to smell the scent of bacon on his clothes. Bacon? That's not normally on Nicky's list of preferred foods, but I figured the other kid's mother must've had some special way of preparing it to get him to eat it, so, very excited, I asked, "How does Pete's mom make it?" Nicky thought about it a moment, then he said, totally innocently, "Like yours. Kind of burned."

I guess Pete's mom burns bacon better than I do.

Eden

schoolteacher

You could be Julia Child, Rachael Ray, Nigella Lawson, Fanny Farmer, and Betty Crocker all rolled into one great big (especially if you eat your own food) cookin' machine, and your kids would still find something to complain about. Or, worse, you could spend twelve years perfecting a recipe for macaroni and cheese, like Michele did, and all they want is Kraft.

Before we get into the recipes, however, we want to address a few food-related issues that many newer mothers confront when their children reach three or four, or even older. The first one is, "Help! My kid won't eat!"

I don't know how to get kids to eat the right foods. My son Jarrod has always liked healthy foods, but my daughter Lucinda has been another story. I will, though, give her credit for improving somewhat on her cheese-based diet that lasted through first grade—it was nothing but mac and cheese, grilled cheese sandwiches, and string cheese—and advancing to chicken, meat, and, *very* occasionally, fish, but she still doesn't like fruit or veggies. So I sneak them in: on Sunday mornings, I'll puree a banana in the Cuisinart and add that to pancake batter (so far she's never noticed); and when I make spaghetti sauce Bolognese, I puree the carrots so that they're undetectable.

Kathryn
homemaker

Don't confuse your child's love for you with whether or not he eats your food. They (almost) never have a damned thing to do with one another. (Just for the record, little Nicky is now sixteen-year-old Nick. He remains skinny as a greyhound but healthy as a horse, stands six feet tall, and scored in the ninety-ninth percentile on the PSAT.) Donna's brother, now in his fifties, was such a notoriously bad eater as a kid that he would sit at the

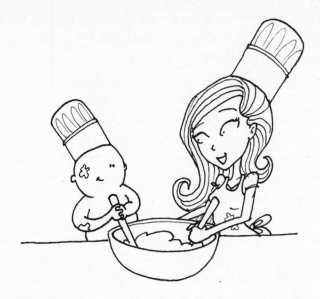

dinner table, count out exactly seven peas, seven tiny pieces of meat, or seven strands of spaghetti, eat only that, and he still grew up superhealthy, with a full head of hair.

Nothin' says lovin' like somethin' from the oven. But it says it even louder when you prepare meals with your kids. This is why we encourage you to get your kids interested in cooking, and it's never too early to start. And should they show a talent for it, why, you just let *them* start preparing dinner, and everybody wins.

It's also never too early to let your kids (and Dad) know that cleaning up is a part of cooking. They won't like it much, but it'll certainly give them a new respect for housework.

The first step to getting them to learn how to cook is for you to cook with them. But it doesn't have to be elaborate, and it doesn't have to be a six-course meal, either.

Don't worry about cooking the entire meal together; buy the entrée ready-made, and have your child help you with the salad. They love drying lettuce in salad spinners (just watch out so they don't spin them right off the counter). Sometimes they also have fun shelling peas, peeling carrots, mashing potatoes, and setting the table.

Here's another clever way to get kids to eat dinner:

Whenever my brothers or I read a book that had a good meal described in it, Mom would cook the meal for us. I'll never forget this one book that my older brother read in fourth grade (that I read in fourth grade several years later), about a kid on a stagecoach. He and his family had been on a long, dusty, bumpy ride, and finally stopped at a way station. Inside was this big meal spread out for them: roast chicken, cherry pies, and mashed potatoes are three things I remember, particularly a passage that talked about the "mountains of mashed potatoes with streams of melted butter running down the sides." I know that there were other dishes described in that chapter, but those are the ones I recall best. So Mom, who is a terrific cook and artist, recreated the meal in perfect, delicious detail.

Joy
editor

Whoa, making a positive association between food and books? Genius, on both counts. You could keep doing it through high school even, although you might draw the line at replicating the fried-dough repast featured in *The Grapes of Wrath* or Miss Havisham's cobweb-draped wedding dinner from *Great Expectations*.

What follow are not only some pointers on getting your child to eat more, and eat better, but several favorite recipes from our kitchens, including some that your kids can make on their own. We hope they, and you, will enjoy them as much as we and our children have.

But Don't Call Me Late for Breakfast

Saturday and Sunday mornings are great opportunities for offering the kids a leisurely, home-cooked breakfast that they can help prepare. But during the school week, most of us are lucky to get out of the house with our teeth buttoned and our clothes brushed—we mean, oh, you know what we mean.

Some breakfast tips:

- Serve precooked bacon that can be heated in the microwave (or fry your own bacon the night before, refrigerate it, then reheat it in the toaster oven in the morning)
- Serve microwaveable oatmeal
- Make smoothies the night before; in the morning, remix them in the blender
- For hot or cold drinks to take in the car, buy to-go hot cups and fill them with hot chocolate, cold juice, or smoothies (Donna refers to this as being your own Starbucks)

Easy Omelets

Crack 2 eggs into a cup and beat very lightly; pour into a quart-size Ziploc bag. Have ready a variety of ingredients, such as grated cheese, ham, crisp bacon, chopped onion, chopped tomatoes, green onions, sliced black olives, etc., to add (assemble these the night before and store in the fridge). Place the ingredients of your choice in the bag, and shake to distribute. Press all the air out of the bag, and zip. Place the bag into boiling water for exactly 13 minutes; up to six bags will fit in a large pot. Open the bag, and the omelet will roll out easily.

Freckled Eggs—Liz Lang

The kale has a mild taste when used in moderation, and the kids get a shot of vegetables without knowing it.

Half a head of kale, washed and thoroughly dried
1 Tbsp olive oil
1 tsp garlic salt

Preheat oven to 300°. Remove stems; chop the kale. Place in a Ziploc bag with the olive oil and the garlic salt, and shake it to coat. Empty the bag onto a cookie sheet in a single layer, and bake till crispy, about 45 minutes. Remove and cool for 10 minutes; then store in a freezer-proof container. When you make scrambled eggs, sprinkle in the kale before the eggs set, about 2 Tbsp kale per 5–6 eggs. Six-year-old William says, "It makes me strong, like Superman!" Says Liz, "If only William could clean up a kitchen like Superman . . ."

Make-ahead Cheese and Sausage Breakfast Casserole— Nicole Fordham

This is also a great dish to assemble on Christmas Eve; pop it into the oven the next morning before you begin opening gifts and it'll be ready before your kids finish complaining about what Santa didn't bring them.

8–10 white bread slices, crusts removed, cut into 1-inch cubes
1 lb. bulk mild breakfast sausage, crumbled and cooked through
1½ cups grated yellow or white cheddar
10 large eggs
2 cups milk
2 tsp Dijon mustard
1 tsp salt
Freshly ground black pepper

Grease a 9″ × 13″ × 2″ glass baking dish. Place the bread in the dish. Top with the meat and cheese. Beat together the eggs with the next three ingredients. Season with the pepper. Pour over sausage mixture. Can be prepared one day ahead; chill. Preheat oven to 350°. Bake until the center is set, 45–50 minutes. Serves 4–5.

The Lunch Bunch

There are two kinds of lunches for kids: the kind you can control (lunch at home), and the kind you only think you control (lunch at school).

Lunch is a food-al area that turns womenfolk into jittery mounds of maternal Jell-O. There's nothing worse than packing your child a nice, wholesome lunch in the morning, then seeing her come home with half of it still in there, all mashed up or dried out. (Actually, there is one thing worse: finding it all squished in her locker six months later.)

But even if her bag, box, or locker is empty, how can you be sure that she ate it all? Easy. If your kid comes home from school ravenous, it means either she didn't eat her lunch because she didn't like what you packed her, or else she did like what you packed her but you didn't pack enough of it. So? Ask her! And if you're not giving her the foods she likes, establish what those foods are. Adults have their own food likes and dislikes; so do kids.

No matter what I'd pack for Travis's lunch, it came back home with him every day. Peanut-butter-and-jelly sandwich? He'd eat half of it. Baloney sandwich? He'd eat the baloney and stick the bread back in the baggie. Apples, grapes, pears? No, let's not even go there. I was about to go insane when one day he came home from school raving about this "really cool" food one of his friends had in his lunch. "Carrots!"

I pointed out that I'd packed him raw carrots about a billion times before, but he never ate them. "Not those kind," he said. "I mean the carrots with the sauce on 'em." So, I found out from the other kid's mom that the "sauce" was ranch dressing. Hidden Valley Ranch? *That's* all it took to make a vegetable lover out of my kid?! Now I pack him raw carrots and a little Tupperware container of HVR every day; and when I recently added raw celery sticks, Travis liked those too. I have no idea how well raw cauliflower will go over, but it's next on my "to sneak in" list.

Gabriela

hair stylist

When in doubt, just throw some Hidden Valley Ranch on it; with most kids, it works every time. They get their veg, their dairy, their herbs . . . it's truly the Wonder Topping. They also love it on chicken nuggets, hamburgers, and what's that other thing you can use it on? Oh, yeah, salad.

Most kids enjoy yogurt for lunch or as a snack; they also like yogurt-based drinks (just make sure to buy the kind that are packed in plastic bottles that won't get squished). Besides fresh fruit, another healthy snack for kids is the Balance bar, which is sweet but nutritious. Chips are not an ideal choice for snacks; they tend to be greasy, and if your child (read, "son") isn't a great one for using that napkin you packed for him, he'll get grease stains on his books and papers.

Another method for getting children to pay more attention to their lunch is to get them a really cool-yet-practical lunchbox (equally important: easy to clean). Some of the snazzier utensils and boxes we've seen lately:

The My Ti Folding Spork from Brunton is a combination spoon and fork with a handle that folds to let it rest compactly inside a lunchbox. Dishwasher-safe ($15, available at www.rei.com).

For a vast variety of tin and plastic lunchboxes, go to www.wicked-coolstuff.com for boxes featuring Supergirl, Spiderman, Batman, Wonder Woman, Betty Boop, Care Bears, Dora the Explorer, Disney characters, Spongebob, et al., starting at $7.95. And for you, Mom, there's even the Sex Pistols lunchbox with drink container, for only $19.95 (just don't pack any Johnny Rotten sandwiches).

There are over a hundred different lunchboxes on display at www.lunchboxes.com. Many of them feature a sandwich box that keeps its contents right-side up; there's even an outside pouch for a cell phone. No kidding ($14.95 and up).

The FUNtainer food jar from Thermos will keep hot foods hot and cold foods cold until your little chow hound adjourns for lunch ($14.99, at www.thermos.com.)

Well-made cloth and reusable plastic lunch bags are available at www.resuablebags.com, starting at $12.95.

It's pricey, but the Laptop Lunch Bento Box lets you easily size your child's food portions in a series of color-coded containers that fit together neatly and elegantly, to ensure against spills ($34.95, at www.reusablebags.com).

To keep cupcakes from losing their icing, try the individual Cup-a-Cake carrier. It's specially designed to hold the cupcake in place even when the lunchbox is turned upside down ($5.95 for a set of two, at www.bakerscatalogue.com).

For homemade lunchbox entrées, our friend Laurie Zaidman offers these suggestions:

- To make shaped sandwiches, remove the crust of soft bread. Build a sandwich with the spread and filling of your choice; lightly press the layers together. Then use a cookie cutter to cut out the desired shape—heart, pumpkin, snowman, etc. Fillings that won't fall out are turkey, smoked salmon, roast beef, cheese, and peanut butter and jelly.
- For vegetarian burritos: warm vegetarian refried beans (make sure they haven't been fried in lard) and spread on a whole-wheat tortilla. Sprinkle shredded low-fat cheese on the beans, and roll it up.

When your child is ready for lunch, and, assuming students have access to a microwave, as many do, she should reheat the burrito on 90% power for about 30–45 seconds.

- Good leftovers for lunch that travel well and may be eaten at room temperature are: penne pasta with pesto sauce; pasta salad with vinaigrette; fried, poached, or roasted chicken; and cold roast beef (fat trimmed).
- For a low-cal, low-fat dessert, spread a whole-wheat, corn, or flour tortilla with a butter/margarine blend. Cut into wedges and sprinkle with cinnamon and sugar. Toast in 350° oven for 2–4 minutes. Wrap in tin foil. Pack it along with a small container of chopped fruit; apples go best.

After you've established what your child is willing to take for lunch, you've got to ask yourself the most important question of all: unless the school has no cafeteria or hot-lunch program (or, if it does and the food is just so horrifically gross that you wouldn't let Sparky eat there, much less your kid), why would you want to pack him a lunch when you can just buy it? Most of the time, the school lunches are cheaper than what it would cost you to send from home; and you won't fall victim to Lunch Stress, not the least of which is having to pack lunch in the morning while you're trying to get yourself and/or your family out the door on time. When they lack the on-campus facilities to serve a hot lunch, many schools make arrangements with their local Subway, Domino's, Pizza Hut, etc., to deliver lunch several times a week. Typically, you pay up-front for the semester, by check.

Jewish Penicillin

When you have a sick child at home, there's nothing better than soup, humankind's oldest recipe. Theory has it that as long as ten thousand years ago, Neanderthals began filling the cleaned, watertight, heatproof hides of animals with meat and water, then suspended them over a fire on forked sticks. Even in the Stone Age, woman had already learned the curative power of soup. And how to be nice to hunters.

Chicken Soup

Michele and Donna prefer kosher chicken, because they find it more flavorful; Ilene prefers regular chicken, because she thinks the kosher birds are too salty. Whichever kind you use, don't skimp on the chicken. There's nothing worse than watery, flavorless soup.

5–7 lbs. kosher chicken
4–5 stalks celery, with leaves on
1 16-oz. bag of peeled baby carrots
1–2 bay leaves
1 large onion, peeled, ends trimmed
3 cloves garlic, peeled, whole
½ tsp salt
1 tsp freshly ground black pepper
Chopped fresh parsley
Fresh dill (optional)

Wash the chicken and pat dry with paper towels; place in a stock pot. Fill the pot with cold water to no more than 2 inches above the chicken. Place the pot on the stove over high heat, with lid off. As water reaches a boil, skim off brown foam that collects; reduce heat to a simmer. Add remaining ingredients, cover, and simmer on very low for at least 2½ hours. Remove the pot from heat and strain the broth, reserving the chicken and carrots. Add carrots back to the strained broth. Add parsley (and dill, if using). Cut up the chicken and return all or some of it to the broth; or else reserve it for chicken salad and sandwiches. Reheat broth just to the boil, and serve with cooked noodles. This recipe makes about 1½ quarts, and can be frozen for up to two months.

If you'd like the soup ready sooner, just substitute canned chicken broth for half of the water (just be sure the chicken is cooked all the way though). The flavor won't be quite as good, but when a little one is sick in bed and needs nourishment fast, it'll taste like ambrosia.

Variations: In addition to the onion, throw in 3 large leeks, sliced ¼″ thick, white part only. For a slightly sweet taste, include one medium-size peeled parsnip with the vegetables; discard after soup is done.

Because When They've Been Good They Don't Want Broccoli

Here are some of our favorite, easy-to-make, kid-friendly desserts.

Bananas Foster

Donna's boyfriend Marc Robinson whips this up for Georgi whenever she has sleepovers.

¼ cup (½ stick) butter

1 cup brown sugar

½ tsp cinnamon

¼ cup banana liqueur (or cognac)

4 bananas, cut in half lengthwise, then halved

¼ cup dark rum (or just more cognac)

4 scoops vanilla ice cream

Combine the butter, sugar, and cinnamon in a flambé pan or skillet. Place the pan over low heat either on an alcohol burner or on top of the stove, and cook, stirring, until the sugar dissolves. Stir in the banana liqueur, then place the bananas in the pan. When the banana sections soften and begin to brown, carefully add the rum.

Continue to cook the sauce until the rum is hot, then tip the pan slightly to ignite the rum. When the flames subside, lift the bananas out of the pan and place four pieces over each portion of ice cream. Generously spoon warm sauce over the top of the ice cream and serve immediately. Serves 4. (If you're worried about kids getting a buzz from the booze, don't; the alcohol burns off.)

Bite-size Cheesecake—Renato Biribin

6 whole graham crackers

6 oz. creamy, spreadable cream cheese (or ricotta, or mascarpone)

12 Hershey's Kisses (or a comparable amount of any brand of semi-sweet chocolate chips, either milk or dark)

Break the graham crackers in half at the seams. Gently spread a spoonful of cream cheese on each cracker. Place a Hershey's Kiss on top of the cream cheese (or, if using chips, spread over the cream cheese). That's it. It's easy, and tastes like a mini–chocolate cheesecake. If you really want to get adventurous, you can spread raspberry or strawberry jam over the cream cheese and then put the chocolate on top. If parent and child don't mind the likelihood of getting a bit messy, melt the chocolate in the microwave before you put it on the cracker.

Dirt Cups

A treat much loved by kids, and guaranteed to make all moms shudder.

    1 4-oz. package chocolate-flavor pudding (requires 8 oz. milk)
    6 Oreo cookies, crumbled (but not crushed)
    18 Gummi worms

Prepare the chocolate pudding as directed on the package. Divide pudding among 6–8 Styrofoam cups and refrigerate for half an hour. Add crumbled Oreo cookies. Refrigerate for another hour. Before serving, place three Gummi worms in cups, pushing them a little bit into the "dirt." Serves 6.

Gingie's Dump Dessert—Diane Lander

"Gingie" was what all the grandchildren called Diane's mom. "Dump desserts" are popular through the South and the Midwest. But why are they called "dump," you ask?

1 4-oz. package pecan pieces
1 20-oz. can crushed pineapple, with juice
1 20-oz. can cherry pie filling
1 8-oz. container Cool Whip (thawed)
1 14-oz. can Eagle brand condensed milk

Because you just dump everything into a large bowl, cover with plastic wrap, stick it in the fridge overnight, and serve for dessert the next evening.

But Don't Eat These . . .

These recipes aren't for eating, but for having fun.

Pretend Play-Doh

1 cup white flour
¼ cup salt
2 Tbsp cream of tartar
1 cup water
2 tsp food coloring
1 Tbsp vegetable oil (*not* olive oil)

Mix flour, salt, and cream of tartar in a medium saucepan. Combine oil, water, and food coloring; add to ingredients in saucepan. Cook over medium heat, stirring, for 3–5 minutes. It's going to look very blobby, but it will turn out correctly. When it forms a ball in the center of the pan, remove and knead on a lightly floured surface. Store in a large Ziploc baggie and dole out to your budding Rodin.

Bubbles

¼ cup liquid dish detergent (neither concentrated nor ultra; Dawn is best)
½ cup water
1 tsp sugar or 3 Tbsp glycerin (available at any drugstore)

Mix in a container with a lid; shake. Dip your bubble-makin' wand into it and blow!

MORE OTHER MOTHERS' TIPS

- If your child likes fried eggs over-medium, but you don't want to break the yolks, put a little water into a lid the same diameter as the frying pan, and cover it. The steam will cook the yolks in a minute or less.
- Want to get Dad to help with the cooking? Put a small TV in the kitchen.
- If the kids are helping you prepare anything fried and/or greasy, put old towels down around the stove and/or counter to absorb spatters.
- For perfect mashed potatoes, heat the milk before adding it to the drained potatoes.
- It's difficult for little kids to butter their own corn on the cob; help them out by buttering a slice of bread and letting them use that instead of a knife.
- If your child takes lunch to school, pack it the night before.
- Try pitas or wraps stuffed with grilled chicken or veggies; soups and salads; and don't forget last night's leftovers. (If your child is a PB&J hound, check your school's peanut-butter policy before you commit anything to bread.)
- When you pack a cold, canned drink in your child's lunchbox, wrap the can in foil or paper towels so that condensation won't wet the bag, napkin, or other foods (a nice, icy-cold drink is also a great way to keep the other foods chilled).
- Pack premoistened towelettes in your child's lunch box; eventually they catch on to handling food with clean hands.
- If your child's after-school activities necessitate packing additional snacks in the morning, look for items that aren't messy and don't require refrigeration, e. g., Pepperidge Farm Goldfish, Chex mix, bananas, dried fruit, Balance bars, small-size rice or popcorn cakes, granola, and mini soft cheeses (such as Bonbel).

IT'S IN THE GROCERY BAG

These are kitchen staples we recommend if there are kids under 12 in the house:

- Milk
- Eggs
- All-purpose flour
- Cake flour
- Sugar
- Confectioner's (powdered) sugar
- Vanilla extract
- Semisweet chocolate for baking
- Bunch of celery
- Bag of peeled baby carrots
- Hidden Valley Ranch dressing (regular or low-fat)
- Sliced cheese (regular or reduced fat)
- Hot dogs
- Chicken tenders
- Chicken bouillon cubes
- Plain bread crumbs
- Pasta: fusilli, rotelli, and farfalline (spirals, curlies, and bowties are much easier for little kids to spear with a fork than spaghetti is)
- A large jar of marinara sauce

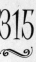

- Hot-dog buns
- Bread
- Mustard, ketchup, and mayonnaise
- Vegetable oil
- Butter, margarine, or reduced-fat butter/margarine blend
- Kraft Easy Mac macaroni and cheese mix
- Canned soups
- Cocoa powder, unsweetened
- Ziploc bags: sandwich, quart, and gallon sizes
- Wine (not to cook with, woman; for your sanity)

Epilogue

Anybody who tells you that raising children is easy is either lying, or has professional help 24/7. On the other hand, raising children is nowhere near as difficult as you fear, and it is our sincere hope that our little book has made that abundantly plain to you.

None of us knew a damned thing we were doing when we brought our tiny babies home from the hospital, but they turned out great anyway.

Marc, twenty-eight, dropped out of college after a sememster, lived on a kibbutz, then came back to the United States to work as a film editor. At twenty-seven he realized he wanted to fulfill his childhood ambition of being a doctor, despite the fact that this was precisely what Michele had always hoped he'd do, and returned to school full-time.

Nikka, twenty-three, majored in musical theater at the Boston Conservatory. After receiving her B.F.A. in 2005, she moved to New York City and has appeared on stage in such productions as *The Who's Tommy* and *Seussical, the Musical.* Okay, so maybe she still hasn't learned how to cook, but the kid orders in like a champ.

Abigail, nineteen, attends college and hopes to become a clinical psychologist, or a fashion designer, or a cosmetics industry tycoon, whichever requires fewer years of school. She shares an apartment with Marc, and marvels that they actually get along, even though he *did* get the bigger bedroom. (No, it never stops.)

And Georgi, fifteen, is a sophmore at Milken Community High School in Los Angeles. She is an accomplished dancer and is involved in numerous school activities. She is interested in everything and capable of anything, and still hugs her mom everyday.

Despite all the worry, the hard work, and the times we wanted to howl at the moon after hearing "Oops, I forgot my science project is due tomorrow," being a mother has been the most rewarding endeavor of our lives. Seeing them walk on those chubby stubbies for the first time, or make the all-star team, or come home with a B+ on the French test they were so afraid they'd *flunkez,* made every sleepless night worth it a million times over.

Motherhood. It's the only job in the world you don't get paid for, your boss is preverbal, and you can't quit.

But the perks are terrific.

Acknowledgments

There are three individuals without whom this book would not have been possible: our superagent, Esther Newberg, who instantly saw our vision and knew exactly what to do with it; our dear friend, Harriet Sternberg, who brought us all together; and our editor, Henry Ferris, whose wit, encouragement, and enthusiasm made the entire experience as smooth as a baby's bottom.

Michele wishes to acknowledge her mother, Sophia McGlade, for her unwaivering love and devotion to the very end of her days; her father, Dr. Frank McGlade, for teaching her "funny"; her brothers, Matt and Marc, for teaching her to fight; her sister-in-law, Karen Caldwell, for her tips and good humor; her cousin, Cathy Stamm, who was her first "other mother" and the best mom in the Greater Philadelphia area; her friend Ursula Zeigler, for her wise and witty stories; her friend Barbara Davilman, for holding her hand and mixing the martinis; and her husband, Andy Guerdat, who's been a far better mother than she could ever hope to be.

Ilene offers her deepest thanks to her husband, Ben Lanzarone, who makes everything possible; to her brother Todd Graff, for his unquestioning help; to her brother Richard Graff and sister-in-law, Lianne, for the laughs and for Holdenn; to her dad, Jerry, and her late mom, Judy, who taught by example . . . living a life of selfless devotion to family and service to those in need; to her aunts, uncles, in-laws, nephews, nieces, and cousins for being the funniest, most loving family; to Donna and Michele for making the dream come true; and to all the special people who helped turn this clueless actress into a pretty decent parent.

And Donna would like to thank her mother, Dorothy, for all her insights, and her father, George, who is reading this book in Heaven with great joy; her brother and sister-inlaw, Les and Norma Rose, and the Golds— Leonard, Barbara, Ethan, and Ilon; her friend Leigh Brillstein, who is always there for her; Rosa Turcios, who is like another mother to Georgi; attorney Mark Temple; friends Mark Pedowitz, Quinn Taylor, Andrea Wong, Kim Fleary, and Jeff Meshel for all their support and guidance; Barbara Lazaroff, Ellen Meyer, Finola Hughes, Karol Pozniak, Marcia Ross, Monica Margalit, Nicky Durlester, Shelly Balloon, Stacey Rosen, and Wendy Devore, who have seen her through everything; Liz Lang, Kendra Castleberry, Marlo Hughling, and Natasha Ward for all their hard work; and Marc Robinson for his love, patience, and wisdom.